Pustules, Pain and Pestilence

Tudor Treatments and Ailments of Henry VIII

Seamus O'Caellaigh

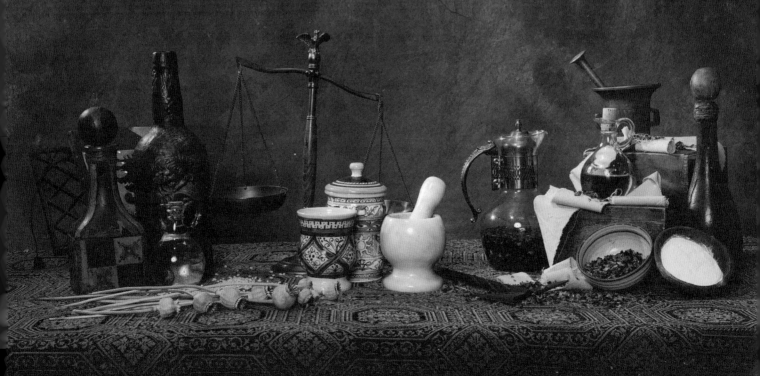

Pustules, Pain and Pestilence:
Tudor Treatments and Ailments of Henry VIII

M
MadeGlobal Publishing

For more information on MadeGlobal Publishing,
visit our website: www.madeglobal.com

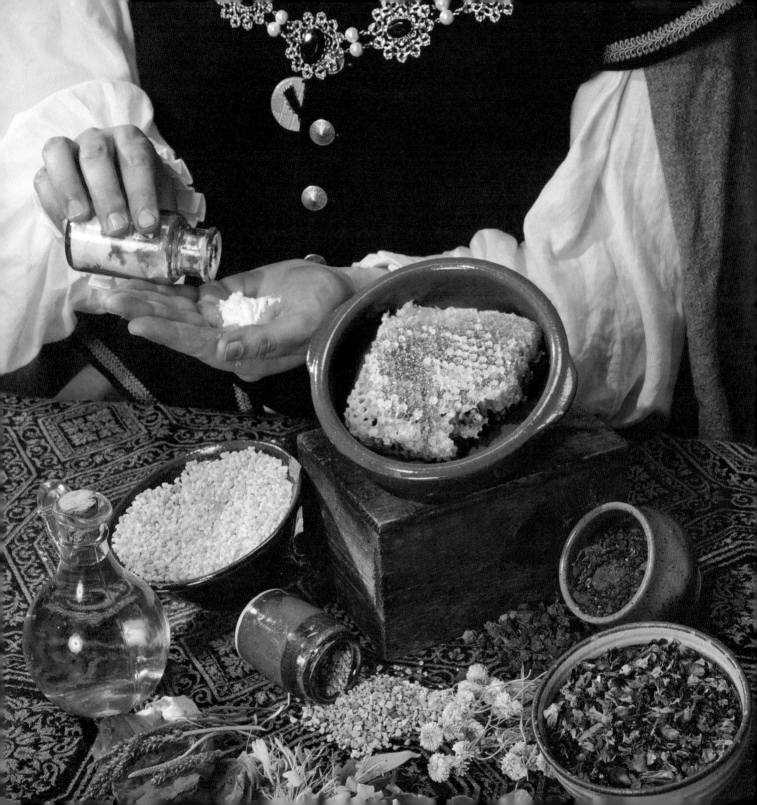

DEDICATION

This glimpse into the world of Tudor medicine is dedicated to a man that has inspired me to take this closer look. David Walddon, you are my mentor and friend, and I would not have started this journey without your support. I cannot think of a person more deserving of this dedication. Your devotion to exploring the pre-16th century life is inspiring and rivalled by few. You have not always been an easy master, but you push where it is needed and do so with love, and I would not have it any other way. A mentor that makes it easy for his apprentice does him no favours.

Thank You
– Your Apprentice

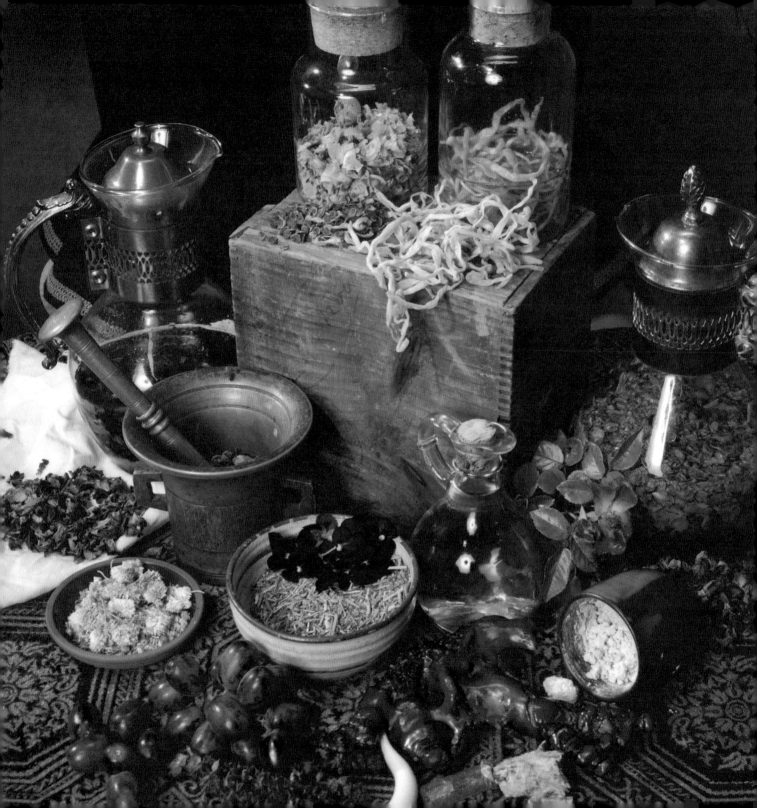

CONTENTS

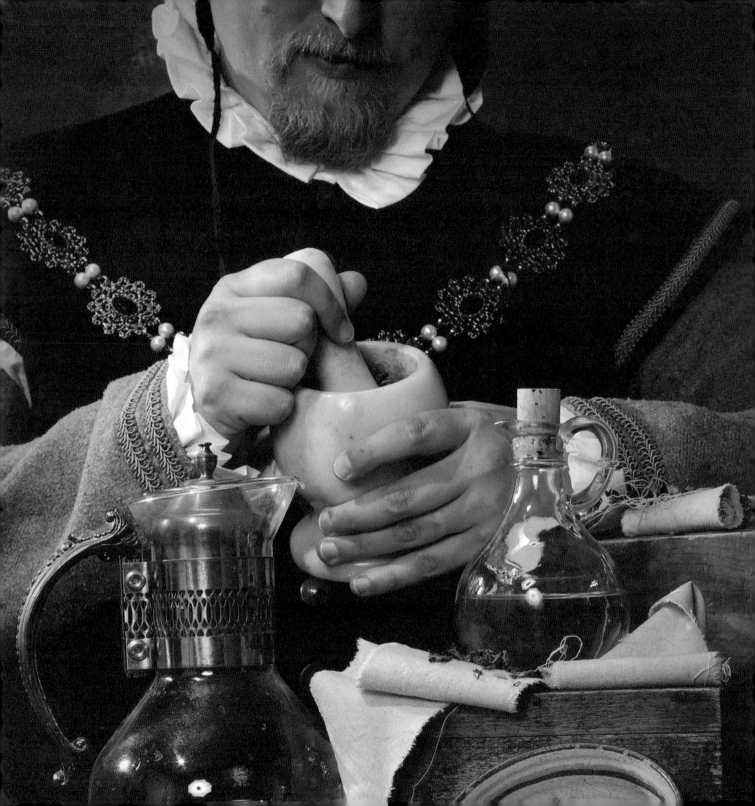

INTRODUCTION

The medical staff of Henry VIII of England left gaps in the medical history of the king. While it is possible that the records have just been lost or destroyed, it is very likely that Henry VIII's physicians did not keep records of what they did to treat Henry, possibly for their own protection. I approached the filling of these gaps by first finding references to his illnesses in letters from his court and from first-hand accounts, recorded in biographies, written by courtiers and staff. Next, I analysed works written by Henry's physicians to determine what Tudor physicians would have done to treat the various illnesses. Using the works of Henry's medical staff, I recreated some of the identified treatments, and I examined the ingredients to look at the history of their uses through early medical texts, and at the harmful effects that could have happened because of our knowledge now of modern medicine and science. This book is a case study, the study of a person over a period of time, not only to present possible treatments for an infamous ruler, but to humanize a science and open a window into the world of Tudor medicine.

LETTERS FROM COURT, DOCTORS, AND MEDICAL TEXTS

The country's future rested heavily on the health of its monarch, so the members of the court, ambassadors, and household members all had their eyes on Henry's health and humours.[1] Through a database of letters from Henry's court, letters from courtiers to their rulers and to each other, and passages in biographies, I found references to many of Henry's illnesses and first-hand accounts of his accidents. These sources revealed two contagious diseases, three accidents that would have had needed treatments, and a slew of medical conditions that troubled Henry until his death.

With the printing press's invention in approximately 1440, herbals[2] and medical texts surged in popularity. Herbals from as early as the 1st century were being published.[3] The availability of so many texts made choosing sources for treatments almost overwhelming. Ultimately, I decided upon only using sources written by Henry's medical staff. Though some were published after the illness or accident happened, I felt they represented a treatment from Tudor England and thus best represented the closest possible treatments for Henry. There are a few treatments that state they were made by His Majesty, but it is unknown if they were made for him to use, if he was involved in their creation, or both.

I started my search for treatments by trying to find "Dr. Buttes' Diary." The diary had been referenced as a source for a leg poultice, made by Dr. Buttes, in the book *The Reign of Henry VIII from His Accession to the Death of Wolsey*. The book written in 1884 by John Murray, said the diary was housed in the British Museum, but after contacting them I found they no longer had a copy of it. I continued looking, and a year into my two-year chase for the diary, historian Steve Bacon appeared as a guest in a documentary; he showed a treatment that he had recreated from a text written by one of Henry's physicians. I found Steve Bacon's contact information and wrote him to see if he knew the location of "Dr. Buttes' Diary" and if that was the text he had used as the source for his poultice recreation. He did not know of the diary's location, but instead pointed me in the direction of *Certaine Workes of Chirurgerie* by Thomas Gale. Thomas was one of Henry VIII's army surgeons and was a dominant figure in the Barber-Surgeons' Guild even into Elizabeth I's reign.[4] Gale's book contains an *enchiridion*, handbook or manual, containing the cures of wounds, fractures, and dislocations, a treatise of the wounds made with gunshot, and a book of antidotes containing the principal and secret medicines used in the art of chirurgerie, as well as some wonderful illustrations of tools used by chirurgeons.

My research also led me to a book written by William Bullein, nurse-surgeon to Henry. William was never admitted into the College of Physicians and the location of his medical degree, if he had one, is unknown. His book *Bullein's Bulwarke of Defense against All Sicknesses, Soreness, and Wounds That Do Daily Assault Mankind: Which Bulwarke Is Kept with Hilarius the Gardener, & Health the Physician, with the Chirurgian, to Help the Wounded Soldiers* was one of the first texts to discuss the sweating sickness that struck London in 1517. It contains: "The Booke of Simples",[5] "A litle Dialogue betweene two men, the one called Sorenes, and the other Chirurgi…", "The Booke of Compoundes",[6] "The Booke of the use of sicke men, and medicines" and even an English theriac recipe.[7]

After reaching out to Elizabeth Lane Furdell, author of *The Royal Doctors 1485-1714*, and the staff at the British Royal Library, I was finally able to find what I had been looking for in the Sloane Manuscript Collection.[8] Over the last 60 years, through various secondary and tertiary sources, it has been called, "Dr. Buttes' Diary," "Prescription Book of Henry," or "Henry's Little Book of Recipes." *Henry VIII of England: Medical receipts devised by the King and the Royal Physicians: 16th century*, is what the British Royal Library calls Sloane Manuscript 1047, a hand-written treasure trove of Tudor Royal Physicians' treatments and recipes.

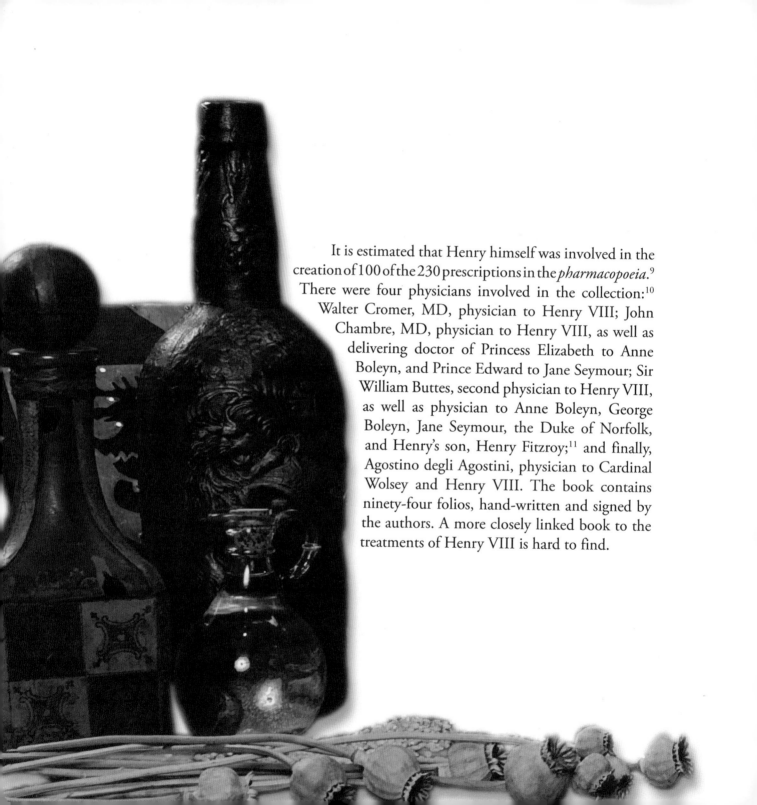

It is estimated that Henry himself was involved in the creation of 100 of the 230 prescriptions in the *pharmacopoeia*.[9] There were four physicians involved in the collection:[10] Walter Cromer, MD, physician to Henry VIII; John Chambre, MD, physician to Henry VIII, as well as delivering doctor of Princess Elizabeth to Anne Boleyn, and Prince Edward to Jane Seymour; Sir William Buttes, second physician to Henry VIII, as well as physician to Anne Boleyn, George Boleyn, Jane Seymour, the Duke of Norfolk, and Henry's son, Henry Fitzroy;[11] and finally, Agostino degli Agostini, physician to Cardinal Wolsey and Henry VIII. The book contains ninety-four folios, hand-written and signed by the authors. A more closely linked book to the treatments of Henry VIII is hard to find.

TUDOR DIAGNOSTIC AND PRESCRIBING TECHNIQUES

To understand the reasoning behind physicians from the 16th century picking a particular treatment, it is important to take a brief look at the theories of the day regarding diagnosing and prescribing. These theories were the tools physicians used to determine what was troubling a patient, as well as what treatment should be used to treat that ailment. Humoral theory, doctrine of signatures, uroscopy and astrological theory were all used in the 16th century to aid a physician. Though modern medicine has found all these invalid, they were commonly used or even required by law into the 1800s.

Humoral theory derives its name from the word humour, meaning fluid. The backbone of the theory is that the body is made up of a mix of four fluids, or humours: black bile, yellow bile, blood and phlegm. When these are out of balance, the patient becomes ill. When a vial of blood is left to sit overnight it can separate into a black clot at the bottom, a red layer of blood cells, a white layer containing white blood cells, and yellow serum at the top. This could very likely be the origins of humoral theory; the black layer thought to be black bile, the red layer the blood, the white layer the phlegm, and the yellow layer yellow bile. Originally associated with Hippocrates in the 4th century BC, humoral theory became common in Europe during the 9th century and was believed to be true into the 1800s. The seasons, climate, diet, occupation, geographic location, planetary alignment, gender, age, and other aspects of a person's life and environment were believed to affect an individual's humour balance. A physician would help a patient rebalance the humours through herbal treatments, based on the plant's quality of moisture and heat, diet, changes to the environment and blood-letting.

Doctrine of signatures, while not named as such until the early 15th century, was used as far back as the 1st century AD. It was suggested in Jakob Böhme's writings that God has marked plants with a sign as to what they are to be used for. The idea is that plants can look like a body part, an animal or be the colour of a humour, and physicians then have a clue as to their proper use. Some examples include: Lungwort being used for lungs due to its spotted leaves that resemble lungs, Eyebright being used for eye ailments due to its eye-like flowers, Great Burnet being red like blood implying that it can be used to balance the humour blood, and Viper's Bugloss having blossoms shaped like a viper's head meaning that it was used to treat viper bites.

Uroscopy is a diagnostic technique that also dates back to Hippocrates in the 4th century BC. Uroscopy is the medical examination of urine to facilitate the diagnosis of a disease. The colour, cloudiness, presence of precipitates or particles, and even the taste of the urine were used to help a physician determine the reason for the patient's illness. A common image of uroscopy in the period's medical text includes around twenty round-bottomed flasks filled with urine of various colours. Urine that is cloudy and milk-like could indicate a urinary tract infection, red like saffron could indicate a problem with the liver, the bacteria pseudomonas could cause green urine, and urine the colour of wine could indicate blood in the urine. There are many illustrations in medical texts of physicians observing the urine of a patient through a crack in a curtained window.

The fourth diagnostic or prescribing practice is medical astrological theory. Medical astrology suggests the association of each sign of the zodiac with parts of the body. The zodiac man was a common illustration in almanacs carried by many physicians and it pointed to the various parts of the body and labelled the zodiac sign that ruled that part. The zodiac man showed that Aries ruled the head, Taurus the neck, Gemini the arms, Cancer oversaw the chest and breasts, Leo the heart and spine, Virgo controlled the digestive system, Libra the kidneys and buttocks, Scorpio governed the reproductive system, while Sagittarius governed the hips and thighs, Capricorn had power over the knees, Aquarius the ankles, and finally Pisces presided over the feet. Ancient studies of astrology were translated from Arabic to Latin in the 12th and 13th centuries and soon became a part of everyday medical practice in Europe. By the end of the 1500s, physicians across Europe were required by law to consult a star chart and calculate the location of the stars before carrying out complicated medical procedures, such as surgery or bleeding.

AILMENTS OF HENRY VIII

Henry VIII lived for 55 years. Henry had many health issues, particularly towards the end of his reign. References to the many accidents and illnesses throughout his life made the choice of what to include difficult. It was not within the scope of this project to include every health issue Henry experienced; the last months of his life, alone, could provide for a lifetime of research. Instead, I decided to include one major accident, two minor accidents, five major illnesses and one minor illness. For these nine ailments, I have included seventeen treatments.

For his bout with smallpox, in 1514, there are four treatments; each addresses a different symptom that comes with the illness. I included a treatment for fever, fitful sleep, pustules, and the scabs that form after the pox. The second illness, tertian fevers, happened in 1521. I included a treatment specifically for tertian or quartan fevers. In 1539, Henry's diet, along with other aspects of his lifestyle, caused him to be very troubled by constipation. It is referenced that he took pills and used a glyster, so I included a recipe for both.

Henry's legs were a major issue and troubled him from 1527 until his death in 1547. His leg issues started with swelling and an ulcer on his left leg. I included a treatment for his swollen legs, a treatment for an ulcer, and a third treatment for the pain. After ten years of regular trouble with his left leg, in 1537 ulcers formed on both his legs. I included a second treatment for ulcers, as well as another for pain. His legs continued to worsen. Later in that year and into the next year, a fistula formed. I have included a treatment for that as well.

Henry had three sporting accidents, two while jousting and one from tennis. His first jousting accident was in 1524. It was relatively minor. He took a lance to the brow, but suffered no lasting damage. For this minor wound, I have included one treatment. Three years later, Henry wrenched his ankle. Though it was a minor accident, it had an effect on the fashion of the court; I included it and two treatments. Nine years later and eager to prove he was still athletic, Henry entered another joust. This accident was the most drastic and life changing of his life. It is often noted as a turning point and blamed for his radical change in mood. He also suffered a leg wound as well as the possible changes in mood due to being knocked unconscious. For the leg wound I have included a wound flush as well as a wound plaster.

Each illness or accident has been given its own section in chronological order. With each ailment are the first-hand accounts, descriptions of the treatments, and, in most cases, a recreation of the treatment or the ingredients. The treatments include a transcription of the original source, as well as the passage being rewritten to fix the Tudor English spelling, and definitions of less common words for ease of reading. The following chapters are a glimpse at Tudor medicine and the king that very well could have received many of these treatments.

1514
SMALLPOX

Many of those interested in the history of the Tudor dynasty know of the *Mary Rose* and her sinking in the Battle of Solent, or at least the treasure trove of artefacts found when she was raised in 1982 from the sea. Not as well-known is the *Henry Grace à Dieu*, another of Henry's ships and the flagship of his fleet. "Great Harry" as the ship was nicknamed was dedicated in the year 1514. According to *Letters and Papers,*[12] Sir Thomas Wyndham and 900 crew members were appointed to the *Grace à Dieu* in 1514. This added to the British Navy the largest war ship in the world, and thus made 1514 a very important year for Henry and his military. However, this was the year that Henry contracted one of the two illnesses that cemented his phobia of disease. This phobia made him renowned for moving court if there was an outbreak of illness, and not allowing an ill courtier to remain in court until they were well over their sickness.

The earliest known, and accurate, reference to smallpox in England dates to 1514, the same year that Henry was likely to have contracted the disease. There is a reference to it earlier, in the 14th century, by the town of Gaddesden, but it is likely that it was incorrectly referenced as smallpox or measles. The reasoning is that the text that references it as "mesles" was the old English word meaning leprous in nature, not a reference to measles or smallpox, which are sometimes confused in medical texts.[13]

LETTERS FROM COURT

On 4 March 1514, Ambassador Dandolo, the Venetian Ambassador to the English Court,[14] wrote to Venice, "The King of England has had smallpox and is cured. He will certainly invade France; but the Flemings apparently are not satisfied with the English."[15] The next day, 5 March, Peter Martyr wrote to Ludovico F. Mendoza, "Lady Margaret has thrown John Emmanuel into prison; it is supposed for speaking against Ferdinand. Henry of England has had a fever; the physicians were afraid for his life, but it ended in the small-pox. He is now well again, and rises from his bed, fierce against France . . . 5 non. Martii 1514."[16]

Henry's constitution and health were praised for his fast recovery. In fact, after only a few days, Henry was out of bed and planning a campaign against France. Not only was there the above correspondence about Henry's illness, later that year a poem was written to Henry about his recovery from the illness.

A NEW-YEAR ODE 1514

(To his Grace King Henry VIII, on his recovery from a fever which threatened small-pox.)

"

If ever noble man where bound to thank god
your grace is most bound for this scourge & rod
for by this scourge is much more comprised
than with head or heart can be devised
by this punishment which seemeth as a cross
better you know god, & yourself never the worse
be simple / Christ saith / as is the pore dove
be wise as the serpent & know whom ye love
be gentile / do justice both to old and young
beware of all flatterers / whereof you had store/
avenge not / reward them / but trust them no more
credit few complaints be they never so strong
have both pity speak so shall you do no wrong
this thing well weighed & your life so directed
shall cause you to live sure though you be suspected
take this in good part / which I for a pow shift
do give unto your grace for a new year's gift.[17]

WHAT IS SMALLPOX?

To understand what treatments could have been used by Henry's physicians, it is important to know the symptoms they would have been faced with treating, and what this disease entailed. "The pox part of smallpox is derived from the Latin word for "spotted" and refers to the raised bumps that appear on the face and body of an infected person."[18] This illness was taken very seriously, until its extermination, because it was often fatal and was easily transmitted. The disease could be spread through direct contact, contact with body fluids, and contact with the bedding or clothes of an infected person. A sufferer could be contagious when the fever started at the beginning of the illness, but were most contagious when the rash appeared. When the rash had started, the infected person was not able to move much and was contagious until the last smallpox scab fell off.

Upon exposure to the virus, an incubation period started. During that time, a person did not exhibit any symptoms and was generally unaware that they had been exposed. This incubation period usually lasted twelve to fourteen days. During the incubation period, people were not contagious. Incubation was over when the first symptoms of smallpox began. The symptoms could include high fever, weakness, head and body aches, and vomiting. This could last for two to four days. After the high fever, spots started to appear in the mouth. "These spots develop into sores that break open and spread large amounts of the virus into the mouth and throat."[19]

When the sores in the back of the throat started to break down, a rash would start to appear on the skin, moving from the face, to the trunk, and then out to the limbs. When the rash started, the fever usually broke and the person may have started to feel better. On the third day of the rash, the rash became the well-known raised bumps that were the disease's namesake. On the fourth day, the bumps began to fill with a thick cloudy fluid. The fever would often rise again and remain high until scabs formed. The bumps felt like there were hard objects inside them, like a bead under the skin. The second week after the rash appeared, most of the sores had scabbed over. "The scabs begin to fall off, leaving marks on the skin that eventually become pitted scars. Most scabs will have fallen off three weeks after the rash appears."[20]

TREATMENTS FROM THE TUDOR PERIOD

For palliative care of symptoms associated with smallpox, I have included four treatments: one for fever, one for the pustules, one to induce sleep when troubled by fever, and one for scabs; all are from William Bullein's book. The first is a treatment made from barley to help temper the fever or "quench hot burning Choler above nature, in vehement fevers." The second is also made from barley and is intended "to reconcile sleep to the afflicted with the fever." The third treatment is a sulphur-based oil for the pox themselves, and in the same passage is the fourth treatment for scabs, a sulphur-based ointment, which could be used to help with the scabs that form over the pox in approximately the second week.

Fever Treatment
- Bullein's Bulwarke of Defence -
William Bullein

"

Now I pray you, what is Barly of nature?

Commonly knowen al this Realme, it is the mother of the best Malt, wherof both Bere and Ale is made: there is Barire double, or with fower set, and syngle two set The greattest and whytest is best, and it is colde and dry in the fyrste degree: and doth not noryshe so muche as Wheate. Of this Barlye, being hulled and clensed from the rynde, beaten or broken, is made the noble drynke called Ptisana: apound beyng put into ten poundes of Cleane water, sodden vnto halfe, into a stone pot, or tynned vessel, close in the mouth, standing vntil it be colde, and then let it runne through a strayner, and so drynk simple of this, for it wil quench hoat burninge Choller aboue nature, in vehe/ment feuers..."[21]

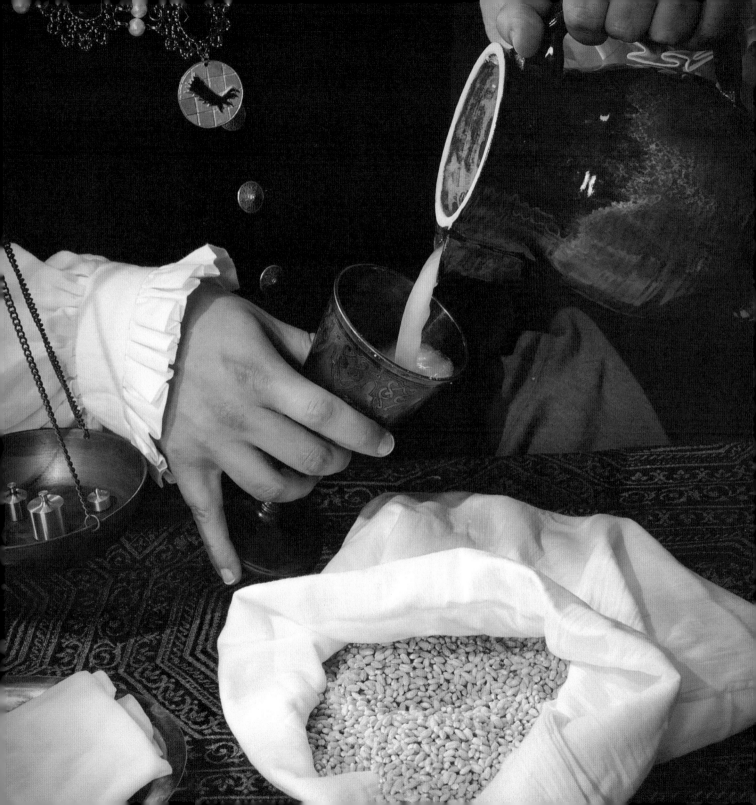

Within this passage, barley water is not only the treatment for fever but also the treatment to help induce sleep, which will be looked at next. I have corrected the spelling to make it easier to read, defined the less common words, and included the likely species of plants. William Bullein wrote this about the nature of barley:

"*Commonly known all this realm, it is the mother of the best malt, where both beer and ale is made: there is barrier double, or with flower set, and single two set. The greatest and whitest is best, and it is cold and dry in the first degree: and doth not nourish so much as wheat. Of this barley, being hulled and cleansed from the rind, beaten or broken, is made the noble drink called Ptisana:[22] around being put into ten pounds of clean water, sodden unto half, into a stone pot, or tinned vessel, closed in the mouth, standing until it be cold, and then let it run through a strainer, and so drink simple of this, for it will quench hot burning choler[23] above nature, in vehement fever.*"

The treatment for fevers says to take barley, hulled and cleaned, and make a drink, called a tisane. To make the tisane, Bullein said to put ten pounds of clean warm or hot water into a stone or tinned vessel pot, and add enough barley to take up half the water, let stand until it's cold, and then strain, and drink. This passage implies that the humour that is out of balance is yellow bile, for it is hot and dry and of a choleric temperament. Humoral theory dictates that this treatment will help stabilize that imbalance.

"

The best barley is white and clean but it is less nourishing than wheat; yet barley water is more nourishing than the polenta that is made of it by reason of the cream that comes off it in the boiling. It is good for irritations, roughness of the arteries and ulcers. Wheat water is also good for these things as it is more nourishing and diuretic. It causes an abundance of milk boiled together with fennel seed and sipped. It is urinary, cleansing, flatulent, bad for the stomach, and ripens oedema. Meal of it boiled with figs, honey and water dissolves oedema and inflammation. It digests hard lumps with pitch, rosin and doves' dung. It brings ease to those troubled with pain in their side with melilot and the heads of poppies. It is applied as a poultice with flax seed, fenugreek and rue against gaseousness in the intestines. With moist pitch, wax, the urine of an uncorrupted child and oil it ripens scrofulous tumours. With myrtle, wine, wild pears, bramble, or pomegranate rinds it stops discharges of the bowels. With quinces or vinegar, it is good for gouty inflammation. Boiled with sharp vinegar (as a poultice made of barley meal) and applied warm it cures leprosy. Juice extracted out of the meal with water and boiled with pitch and oil is good for discharges of the joints. Meal of barley stops discharges of the bowels and lessens inflammation.

Dioscorides[24]

SLEEP AID
- BULLEIN'S BULWARKE OF DEFENCE -
WILLIAM BULLEIN

"

...You may put in the Seedes of whyte Poppy, and Lettice not onely to coole, but also to reconsyle sleape to the afflicted with the Feuer to clense corruption of the Lunges, and horsenesse, with shortnesse of wynd Put in Figges, Liquoris, Annisseedes, Reysynges of the Sun, and a little Hysope with Suger: seeth al, and let it stand close vntill it bee colde, and strayne it wyth a strayner, and so drynke therof, for the foresayd shortnesse of wynde. Seeth Barly meale, Lint seede, and Fenegreke seede, and the iuice of Rew with Malmesye, warme applyed to the belly, wil put awaye swellyng and paynes in the guttes. The meale therof sodden in vineger, wil asswage the hoate burnyng goute: and this is good agaynst all hoate inflamations of the body. And seeth Barly in Hony, Rosen, and the iuice of Chelidon, and it wil heale an old rotten sore. With Oyle and Fenegreeke, meale. it wil asswage the swelling of the precordal or stomacke. Melilote, Poppy and Hony tempered togeather, do helpe the swellynge heate of the Priuy members, paynes of the sydes or Flesh, which is gone from ye bone with many other goodly vertues, which Barly hath as affyrmeth .

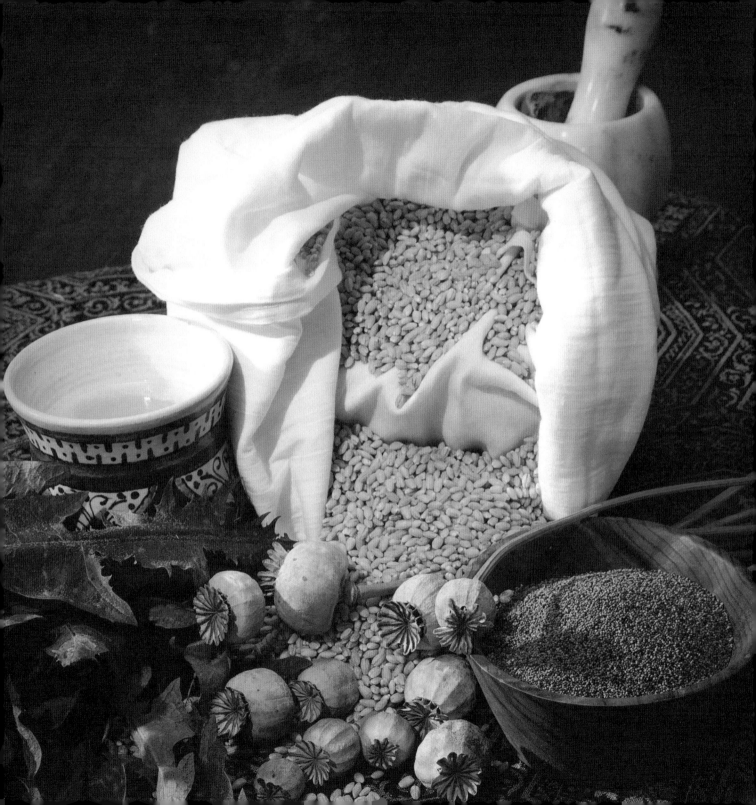

"You may put in the seeds of white poppy, and lettuce not only to cool, but also, to reconcile sleep to the afflicted with the fever, to cleanse corruption of the lungs, and hoarseness, with shortness of wind. Put in figs, licorice, aniseeds, raisins of the sun, and a little hyssop[26] with sugar: seethe all, and let it stand closed until it be cold, and strain it with a strainer, and so drink thereof, for the aforesaid shortness of wind. Seethe barley meal, linseed, and fenugreek seed, and the juice of rue[27] with malmsey,[28] warm applied to the belly, will put away swelling and pains in the guts. The meal thereof sodden in vinegar, will assuage the hot burning gout: and this is good against all hot inflammations of the body. Seethe barley in honey, rosin[29], and the juice of celandine,[30] and it will heal an old rotten sore. With oil and fenugreek, meal it will assuage the swelling of the precordial[31] or stomach. Melilot,[32] poppy, and honey tempered together, do help the swelling heat of the privy members, pains of the sides, or flesh which is gone from the bone with many other good virtues, which barley has as affirmed."

Often with fevers comes the inability to sleep, or a fitful sleep. I included this particular treatment because it used the tisane as a base. If a large batch of the tisane was made to treat the fever throughout the day, a portion could be set aside for a dose at night with extra ingredients included to treat insomnia. William Bullein wrote that putting the seeds of white poppy and lettuce into the tisane would bring sleep to a patient with the fever.

Upon first reading the passage in Bullein's book, it is not surprising to see poppy involved in a sleeping treatment, as it is the plant from which opium is derived. It was also used for other ailments, around 60 AD Dioscorides wrote in *De Materia Medica,*[33] "The heads are boiled alone in water until half, and then boiled again with honey until the dullness is thickened, make a licking medicine soothing for coughs, dripping fluids in the throat, and abdominal afflictions."[34] It might be surprising to see lettuce included. However, with further research I determined that Bullein was not referencing common lettuce. The ingredient William Bullein was calling for is in fact wild lettuce[35] and it was used as far back as the first century.

Dioscorides wrote, "Wild lettuce is similar to the cultivated only larger stalked, paler in the leaves, thinner and sharper, and bitter to the taste. It is somewhat similar to poppy in properties."[36] The whole wild lettuce plant contains a milky juice that emerges when the cuticle[37] is punctured or cut. This juice is bitter and has a foul odour. When the juice dries, it hardens, turns brown, and the resin is called *lactucarium*. When the chemicals in wild lettuce have been studied they have been found to contain lactucic acid, lactucopicrin, lactucerin (lactucone) and lactucin. Lactocerine is the main ingredient that is present in the resin. "Lactucarium is a diuretic, laxative and sedative agent which relieves dyspnoea, and decreases gastrointestinal inflammation and uterus contractions. It has anticonvulsant and hypnotic effects as well. In addition, the lettuce contains traces of hyoscyamine, which is probably responsible for its sedative effects."[38] Both wild lettuce and poppy have been used for over 2,000 years to induce sleep, and with modern science we can see why it was used repeatedly.

PUSTULE TREATMENT
- BULLEIN'S BULWARKE OF DEFENCE -
WILLIAM BULLEIN

"

What is the nature of Sulpher, called Brimstone?

SVLPHER called Brimstone, is hoat and dry in the fourth degree: with this Sulpher, and fyre, God plaged the People of Sodom, and Gomor, for their abhominable Sinnes against Nature. Supher is one of the simples put into the receypt of Gunpouder, wherewyth God by his instruments hath plaged the proude World with, through mercilesse Gunnes, Sulpher is found in diuers partes of ye worlde, as in vaynes of the Earth, Welles, Pittes, aswell in the colde partes of Iseland, as in the hoat partes of Inde. Of a sulpherous humour it is presupposed that the waters of the Bathes heere in England haue their continuall warmnesse. Also in Italy in the fielde Senensis, vpon ye mountaines not farre from the warme Bathes of S. Philip, is mutch Brimstone foūde, therefore it is none errour to say that the hoat Bathes haue their originall spryng of Brimstone. Sulpher hath vertue to dry vp Scabbes being tempred wyth fasting spittle, Uinegar, and Swynes grease. It also helpeth Leprous, Scabbes, and Poxes, being sodden in Oyle Debay, and sharpe Uinegar"[39]

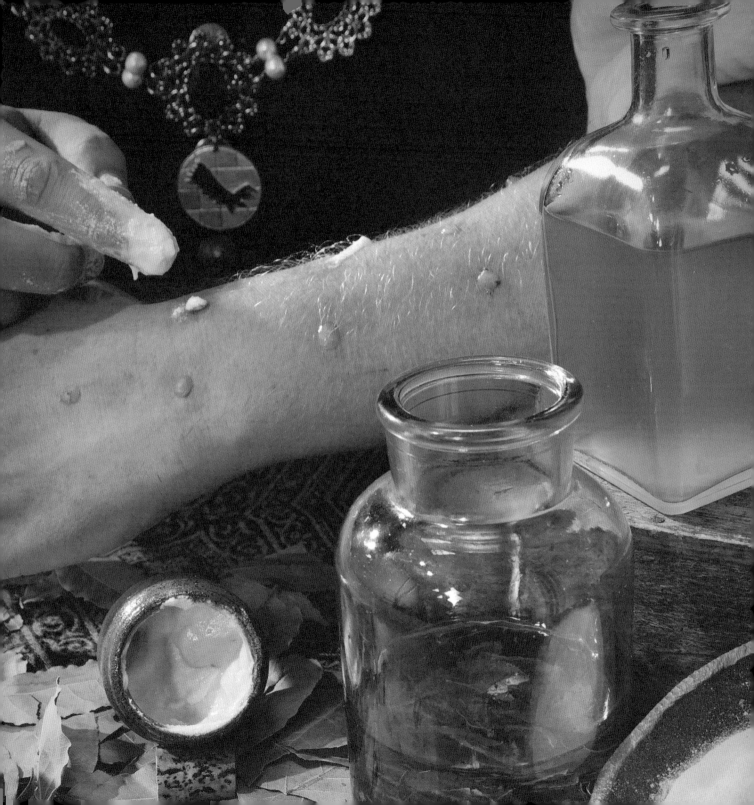

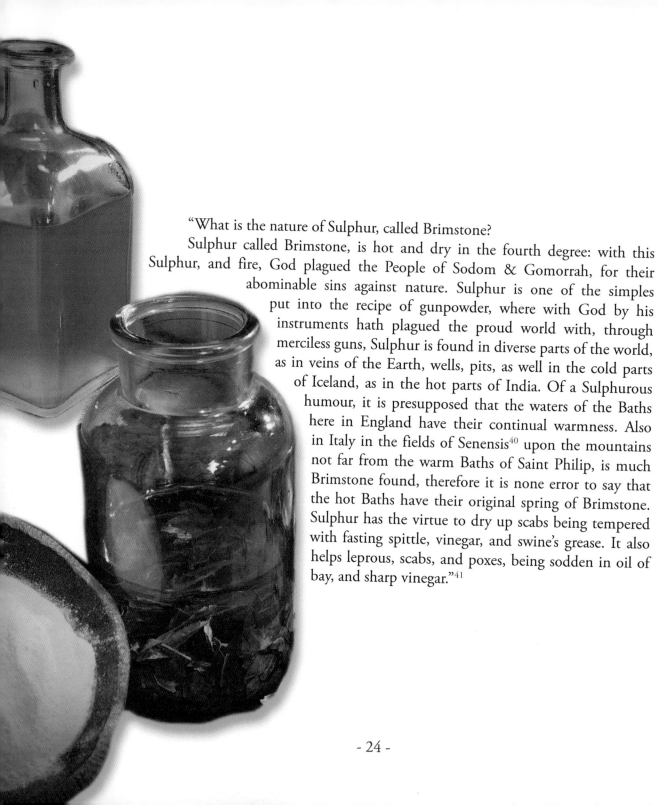

"What is the nature of Sulphur, called Brimstone?

Sulphur called Brimstone, is hot and dry in the fourth degree: with this Sulphur, and fire, God plagued the People of Sodom & Gomorrah, for their abominable sins against nature. Sulphur is one of the simples put into the recipe of gunpowder, where with God by his instruments hath plagued the proud world with, through merciless guns, Sulphur is found in diverse parts of the world, as in veins of the Earth, wells, pits, as well in the cold parts of Iceland, as in the hot parts of India. Of a Sulphurous humour, it is presupposed that the waters of the Baths here in England have their continual warmness. Also in Italy in the fields of Senensis[40] upon the mountains not far from the warm Baths of Saint Philip, is much Brimstone found, therefore it is none error to say that the hot Baths have their original spring of Brimstone. Sulphur has the virtue to dry up scabs being tempered with fasting spittle, vinegar, and swine's grease. It also helps leprous, scabs, and poxes, being sodden in oil of bay, and sharp vinegar."[41]

Bullein also described treating the pox themselves with sulphur sodden in oil of bay and vinegar. The salve was applied to the pox directly. There are two possible ways oil of bay could be made, as a simple oil or a compound oil. Thomas Culpeper, English botanist, herbalist and physician, explains the difference between simple and compound oils.[42] Simple oils are made by pressing fruits or nuts to expel their oil. Compound oils are made with a simple oil, such as olive oil, absorbing the "virtues" of the leaf through the warming of the oil and leaf mixture. Culpeper also wrote about the uses of bay in his herbal, "A bath of the decoction of the leaves and berries, is singularly good for women to sit in, that are troubled with the mother, or the diseases thereof, or the stoppings of their courses, or for the diseases of the bladder, pains in the bowels by wind,[43] and stopping of urine."[44] A simple oil made from the fruit would be stronger and more potent, but if it was not available, a compound oil made with the leaves would be another option.

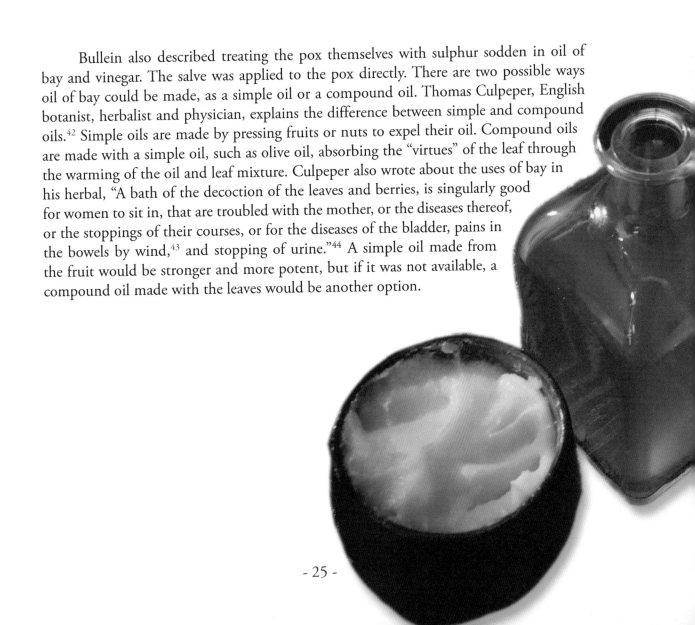

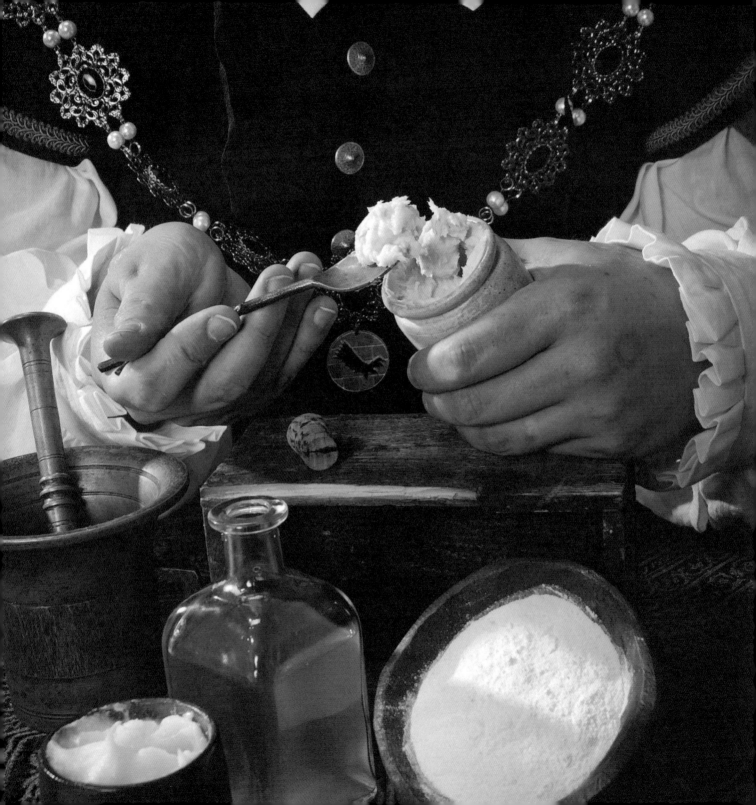

SCAB TREATMENT
- BULLEIN'S BULWARKE OF DEFENCE -
WILLIAM BULLEIN

To help the scabs that formed, Bullein said, "Sulphur hath virtue to dry up scabs" if mixed with fasting spittle, vinegar, and swine's grease. In *De Materia Medica*, "It is also good for gangrenous ulceration, erysipelas,[45] shingles, psoriasis, lichen,[46] and pterygium[47] mixed with some other medicine from those that are suitable."[48] The use of vinegar to fight infections dates back to Hippocrates (460-377 BC). Hippocrates recommended a vinegar preparation for cleaning ulcers and sores.[49] Sulphur was used for various skin conditions, as early as the 1st century, including "leprosy, rotten nails, and itching."[50] Pliny the Elder wrote in his encyclopedia of Roman life, *A Natural History*, that fasting spittle is used to treat "lichen and leprous spots."[51] All three ingredients were used as early as the 1st century, if not earlier, so it is no wonder that Tudor doctors continued to use them through the 16th century and used them in combination to treat scabs on their patients.

These four treatments for the symptoms associated with smallpox show not only what Tudor physicians did to treat the symptoms, and possibly what could have been used to treat Henry VIII, but that medicine of the period drew heavily on the works of earlier physicians. The four treatments; one for fever, one for the pustules, one to induce sleep when troubled by fever, one for scabs; are all from William Bullein's work. The treatment made from barley was used to help temper the fever by balancing the humours with a cool treatment. The second is also made from barley, but with poppy and wild lettuce added to induce sleep. The third treatment is a sulphur-based oil for the pustules formed by the disease, and in the same passage is the fourth treatment, a sulphur-based ointment to use on the scabs that formed over the pox in approximately the second week. Seven years later, Henry would face the second disease that could have been the final nail in the "coffin" of his phobia.

1521
TERTIAN FEVERS

Edward Stafford, 3rd Duke of Buckingham, along with other nobility, had grown to resent Cardinal Wolsey, Henry VIII's advisor. Wolsey had been born to a butcher and his wife, and some of the nobility resented the influence a low-born man had with the king. In 1520, Wolsey received an anonymous letter accusing the Duke of Buckingham of treason, and when Henry heard of the letter he took the charge seriously. Wolsey's supporters had Buckingham tried for treason. The charges were listening to prophesies of the king's death and of his succession to the crown, and expressing an intention to kill Henry VIII. He was taken to the Tower on 16 April 1521. Richard Pace wrote to Wolsey on the same day, "My lord of Durham would have come unto your grace, but the king would not suffer him so to do, but commanded him to tarry here for the examination of certain things of Buckingham's servants. My said lord sendeth unto your grace a letter written by the king's commandment to such as shall see to the charge of the said Duke's house during his absence."[52]

Six days later, the ambassador to the French court, William FitzWilliam, who would later become the first Earl of Southampton, wrote to Cardinal Wolsey, "The French king told me my lord of Buckingham was in the Tower, and asked if I had heard of it. I said, no. He asked me what sort of a man he was. I said I thought he was a high-minded man, and a man that would speak sometimes like a man that were in a rage. And he said he judged him for such a man, and so full of choler that there was nothing could content him. Then I showed him the king's grace had given him good lessons... and so good that, and had he had any grace, he would not have deserved to have been there. And he said it was honorably done of the king's grace to give him warning; and then I showed him I knew his grace had given him warning, as well by your grace as by his own... oftener than once; he praised that very much."[53] At Westminster, on 13 May, Buckingham was tried before a panel of seventeen peers, but with the king's mind already decided, it was unlikely that anything said in the trial could have saved him. The treason statute in effect at the time required overt acts for conviction, nonetheless, Buckingham was found guilty of treasonous speech. Despite a plea for mercy from Queen Katherine of Aragon, he was executed at Tower Hill on 17 May 1521. It was a within a few days that Henry contracted malaria, but his phobia started years before.

Henry's phobia started with the death of his father. The elegy[54] of Henry VII (Composition Date: 1509):

O wavering world all wrapped in wretchedness
What avails thy pomps so gay and glorious
Thy pastimes thy pleasures / and all thy riches
Syth [since] of necessity they be but transitorious
Example but late o to much piteous
The puissant prince that each man whylom [once] dread
Maugre [in spite of] thy might by natural line and course
Henry the seventh alas alas lyeth dead

O case Wonderful so royal a king
Surmounting in manner the prudent salmon
In Wisdom in Riches and in everything
None to him like in no Christian region
Redoubted and feared not long agone
Lauded and praised his name by fame spread

From Worldly content now destitute alone
For henry the seventh alas alas lyeth dead

Lo mark we this matter we wretched creatures
For all his kingdoms and triumphant majesty
For all his joys his pastimes and pleasures
He is now gone without remedy
The soul Where god will the miserable body
Closed in stone and in heavy lead
O what is this world but vanity and all vanity
For henry the seventh alas alas lyeth dead

Come we therefore his subjects and make lamentation.
For the loss of one so noble a governor
To god with our prayers make we exclamation
His soul forto guide to his supernal tower
For faded is the goodly rose-flower
That Whilome [once] so royally all about spread
Death hath him mated where is his power
Henry the seventh alas alas lyeth dead

Of this most Christian king in us it lyeth not
His time-passed honour sufficient to praise
But yet though that thing invalue [place a value on] we may not
Our prayers of surety he shall have always
And though that atropose hath ended his days
His name and fame shall ever be dread
As far as Phoebus spreads his golden rays
Though henry the seventh alas alas lyeth dead

But now what remedy he is uncoverable
Touched by the hands of god that is most just
But yet again a cause most comfortable
We have Wherein of right rejoice we must
His son on live in beauty force and lust
In honour likely Traianus to shed [rout, put to flight]
Wherefore in him put we our hope and trust
Syth [since] henry his father alas alas lyeth dead

And now for conclusion about his hearse
Let this be graved for endless memory
With sorrowful tunes of Thesyphenes verse
Here lyeth the puissant and mighty henry
Hector in battle Ulysses in policy
Solomon in wisdom the noble rose red
Croesus in riches Julius in glory
Henry the seventh engraved here lyeth dead.[55]

The above elegy about Henry VII was written in the year 1509, the year he died of consumption.[56] This was not the only death in Henry VIII's early life, seven years earlier he lost his brother, Arthur, Prince of Wales, to what was likely sweating sickness[57] or consumption. It was said a malign vapour had risen from the marches around Ludlow Castle. This follows with the Tudor belief that many illnesses were caused by bad air that entered the body through the nose or mouth. As we already, know Henry VIII had an attack of smallpox only a few years into his reign. In 1521, his phobia was cemented into place when the king contracted a series of fevers that recurred, today this illness is known as malaria.

LETTERS FROM COURT

Cardinal Wolsey wrote on 20 May 1521 to Sir Richard Jerningham of the king's fever, "As the king did not, at the departure of you Sir Richard Jerningham from hence, write to the French king according to his original intention, you shall both explain to him the cause; viz., that he had just caught a fever, which shortly grew to two tertians. Owing to the long continuance of paroxysms in cold and heat, with no interval between to enable him to take his meals, the physicians were fain to give him his meals before the end of his paroxysms. The disease is now gone, and for five or six days he has been fresh, merry and well at ease; much better than before."[58]

By 24 May, letters started arriving at court, enquiring of the king's health. Francis I of France wrote, "…but hearing that you were unwell I have put aside all other things to send you Montpesat, whom you know, by whom I beg you to send me news of your health. As to the despatch of the said Jerningham I will despatch him in two days, and with him the sieur De la Batye, hoping you will be satisfied. I beg you will send back Montpesat as soon as possible, that I may hear how you are."[59]

The next day, on 25 May 1521, more letters arrived. Bishop Bonnivet wrote to Henry VIII, "My master, hearing you were ill of a fever, sends the bearer, le sieur de Montpesat, to ask after your health." He then wrote to Cardinal Wolsey, "My master hears that the king is ill of a fever, and sends over the bearer, the sieur de Montpesat, a gentleman of his chamber, to ask about his health. He will not be at ease till he is told of his recovery, and is also grieved to hear of your long illness. Jerningham will be despatched in a couple of days, and la Bastye with him, by whom you will receive an ample answer to Jerningham's chares, which will content your master."[60]

WHAT IS MALARIA?

Following an infective bite by a mosquito, the incubation period varies from seven to 30 days. When the disease leaves the incubation period and becomes active, it only lasts for about six to ten hours. These active stages consist of three phases: a cold phase, sensation of cold, shivering; a hot phase, fever, headaches, vomiting; and finally, a sweating phase, sweats, and a return to normal temperature. The attacks occur every third day with the "tertian" parasites (*plasmodium falciparum*, *plasmodium vivax*, and *plasmodium ovale*) and every fourth day with the "quartan" parasite (*plasmodium malariae*). The symptoms are often confused with the flu or a cold.[61]

TREATMENT FROM THE TUDOR PERIOD

I chose a treatment that was used to battle both tertian and quartan fevers, though, as stated in the letter cited above from Cardinal Wolsey, Henry suffered from tertian fevers. This means he was infected by *plasmodium falciparum*, *plasmodium vivax*, or *plasmodium vale*. The treatment is from Bullein's book. In some severe cases, haemoglobin can be destroyed and this can cause the urine to turn dark brown. In the physicians of Myddfai's medical text, the section regarding uroscopy describes what dark and turbid[62] urine means for a patient: "If the urine is dark, during the heat of the fever, the turbidity not subsiding, his illness will resolve itself info an ague in four, or perhaps three days."[63]

Tertian Fevers Treatment
- Bullein's Bulwarke of Defence -
William Bullein

"

Giloflowers are sweete and pleasaunt, but are they good for any medicine?

Yea forsooth, they are no lesse profitable, than pleasaunt, and greatly commended among the olde Wryters: for Dioscorides reporteth of them, that they do not only preserue ý bodies of men from corrupt Ayres, but also keepe the mynde and spyrituall partes, from terrible and fearefull dreames: through their heauenly sauour, and most sweete pleasaunt odour, they do fortifie the brayne: there is no Apothicary can by any naturall Arte, make any confection so pleasaunt as this is, whych nature hath wrought most wonderous in pleasing of the senses, both of seeing and smelling. If Gilloflowers be stamped, they heale newe woundes of ý head, and drawe forth broken bones. The decoction of them is good to washe the head withall. The Oyle of Gillofloures doth heale the byting of a mad dog, and woundes of the sinewes, and cold goutes. If this flower be sodden in whyte Wyne, it driueth away the terrour of a Tertian, and the horrour of a Quarten, being drunke warme before the fit: and by ý meanes also be Wormes killed in the belly. This herbe of nature is hoat and dry..."

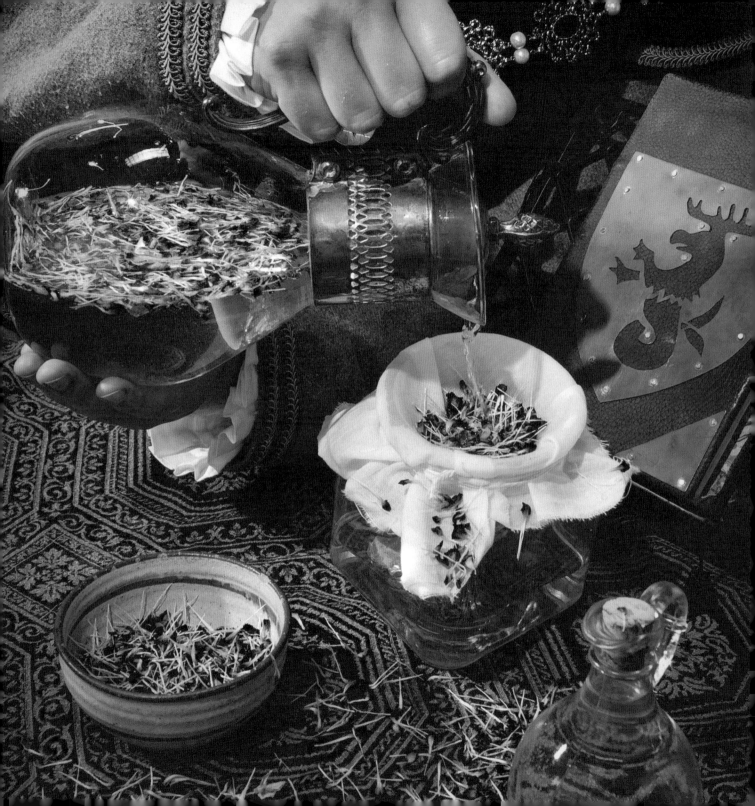

"Gillyflowers are sweet and pleasant, but are they good for any medicine?

Yea forsooth, they are no less profitable, than pleasant, and greatly commended among the old Writers: for Dioscorides reported of them, that they do not only preserve the bodies of men from corrupt airs, but also keep the mind and spiritual parts, from terrible and fearful dreams: through their heavenly flavour, and most sweet pleasant odour, they do fortify the brain: there is no Apothecary can by any natural art, make any confection so pleasant as this is, which nature hath wrought most wondrous in pleasing of the senses, both of seeing and smelling. If Gillyflowers be stamped, they heal new wounds of the head, and draw forth broken bones. The decoction of them is good to wash the head withal. The oil of gillyflowers[65] doth heal the biting of a mad dog, and wounds of the sinews, and cold gouts. If this flower be sodden in white wine, it drives away the terror of a tertian, and the horror of a quarten, being drunk warm before the fit: and by the means also, be worms killed in the belly. This herb of nature is hot and dry…"

If the flowers of the gillyflower are soaked in white wine and drunk warm before the fever comes again, "it drives away the terror of a tertian, and the horror of a quarten." This means the drink would have not been given until the first fever breaks. Gillyflower is a common name for various flowers. Just as the botanists of the time were starting to find out, a common name for some plants could mean multiple species of plant, depending on time and location.

It was written in the beginning of *De Historia Stirpium,* written in 1542 by Leonhart Fuchs, that medicine of the time needed to be mended. He said that physicians were unfamiliar with more than a few herbs and their names, apothecaries only knew some of the plants, and the suppliers of the plants that apothecaries used were uneducated and didn't know the same names as the medical professionals. I chose carnations as the plant I used to recreate the treatment because of the reference to "gillofloures" in Gerard's Herbal. *The Herbal or, General History of Plants* was published in the late 1500s and was written in England, like *Bullein's Bulwarke.* It also includes detailed woodcuts as references, which depict carnations, and the passage names them with both common names. Further support for the selection of carnations can be drawn from Gerard's reference to their use in treating fevers.[66] He also says that they are temperate in temperature which will help to counter the heat of a fever. Once again, the choice in the plant used to treat a fever is due to the belief that a cooling plant will balance the humours. The patient has too much blood or yellow bile, both being warm, and thus the gillyflower will cool that heat and stop the fever.

Tertian fevers were the second disease Henry became infected with, and in three years he would again be under the watchful eyes of his physicians. However, this time it would not be for a contagious disease, but for the first in a series of accidents. His first accident was during a hastilude,[67] a favourite pastime of Henry's, though he loved most physical games and activities. Henry was less interested in running a country early in his reign and even wrote a song about his love of pastimes. "Pastime with Good Company" is an inside look at Henry's love of fun and good sport, and an appropriate transition into the first accident he had while pursuing this love.

"

Pastime with good company
I love and shall unto I die;
Grudge who list, but none deny,
So God be pleased thus live will I.
For my pastance
Hunt, song, and dance.
My heart is set:
All goodly sport
For my comfort,
Who shall me let?

Youth must have some dalliance,
Of good or ill some pastance;
Company methinks then best
All thoughts and fancies to dejest:
For idleness
Is chief mistress
Of vices all.
Then who can say
But mirth and play
Is best of all?

Company with honesty
Is virtue vices to flee:
Company is good and ill
But every man hath his free will.
The best ensue,
The worst eschew,
My mind shall be:
Virtue to use,
Vice to refuse,
Shall I use me. [68]

1524
FIRST JOUSTING ACCIDENT

It is well known that France, England, and Spain throughout the Tudor Period, and in fact before and after, switched sides in who were allies and who they were at war with. The Peace of Étaples in 1492 ended a war between France and England. Then the Treaty of Westminster, in 1511, allied England and Aragon[69] against France, until the Treaty of London which formed a non-aggression pact between Burgundy, England, France, the Holy Roman Empire, the Papacy, Spain, and the Netherlands. In 1522, the Treaty of Windsor was signed between England and the Holy Roman Empire. The treaty charted a combined English-Imperial attack against France, with each kingdom promising to provide at least 40,000 men. To strengthen the alliance, Emperor Charles V also agreed to marry Henry's daughter, Princess Mary. The next year, things started to fall apart for the English foothold in France, even with the looting of the country in Brittany and Picardy. In 1524, England and Charles V supported Charles III, the Duke of Bourbon, in his claim and helped him capture parts of France, sending him men and money.

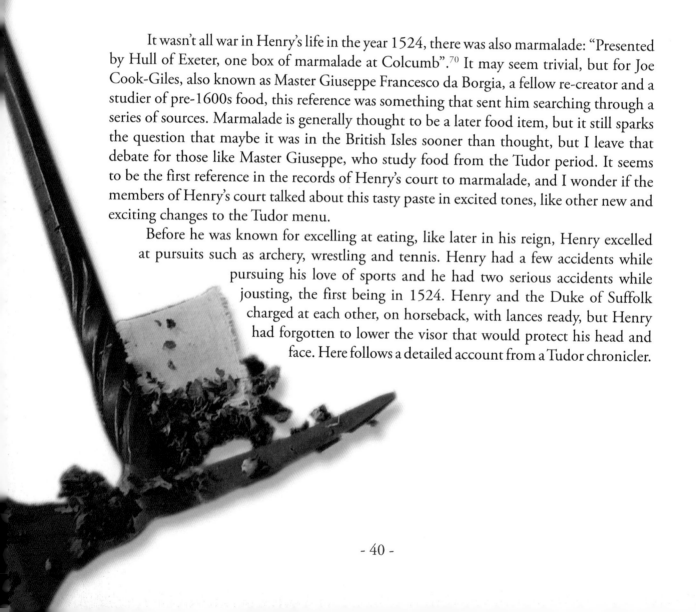

It wasn't all war in Henry's life in the year 1524, there was also marmalade: "Presented by Hull of Exeter, one box of marmalade at Colcumb".[70] It may seem trivial, but for Joe Cook-Giles, also known as Master Giuseppe Francesco da Borgia, a fellow re-creator and a studier of pre-1600s food, this reference was something that sent him searching through a series of sources. Marmalade is generally thought to be a later food item, but it still sparks the question that maybe it was in the British Isles sooner than thought, but I leave that debate for those like Master Giuseppe, who study food from the Tudor period. It seems to be the first reference in the records of Henry's court to marmalade, and I wonder if the members of Henry's court talked about this tasty paste in excited tones, like other new and exciting changes to the Tudor menu.

Before he was known for excelling at eating, like later in his reign, Henry excelled at pursuits such as archery, wrestling and tennis. Henry had a few accidents while pursuing his love of sports and he had two serious accidents while jousting, the first being in 1524. Henry and the Duke of Suffolk charged at each other, on horseback, with lances ready, but Henry had forgotten to lower the visor that would protect his head and face. Here follows a detailed account from a Tudor chronicler.

A Narrative from Court

Chronicler Edward Hall wrote a detailed account:

"

The 10th day of March, the king having a new harness [armour] made of his own design and fashion, such as no armourer before that time had seen, thought to test the same at the tilt and appointed a joust for the purpose.

On foot were appointed the Lord Marquis of Dorset and the Earl of Surrey; the King came to one end of the tilt and the Duke of Suffolk to the other. Then a gentleman said to the Duke, "Sir, the King is come to the tilt's end." "I see him not," said the Duke, "on my faith, for my headpiece takes from me my sight." With these words, God knoweth by what chance, the King had his spear delivered to him by the Lord Marquis, the visor of his headpiece being up and not down nor fastened, so that his face was clean naked. Then the gentleman said to the Duke, "Sir, the King cometh."

Then the Duke set forward and charged his spear, and the King likewise inadvisedly set off towards the Duke. The people, perceiving the King's face bare, cried "Hold! Hold!", but the Duke neither saw nor heard, and whether the King remembered that his visor was up or not few could tell. Alas, what sorrow was it to the people when they saw the splinters of Duke's spear strike on the King's headpiece. For most certainly, the Duke struck the King on the brow, right under the defence of the

cont.

headpiece, on the very skull cap or basinet piece where unto the barbette is hinged for power and defence, to which skull cap or basinet no armourer takes heed of, for it is evermore covered with the visor, barbet and volant piece, and so that piece is so defended that it forceth of no charge. But when the spear landed on that place, it was great jeopardy of death, in so much that the face was bare, for the Duke's spear broke all to splinters and pushed the King's visor or barbet so far back by the counter blow that all the King's headpiece was full of splinters. The armourers for this matter were much blamed and so was the Lord Marquis for delivering the spear when his face was open, but the King said that no-one was to blame but himself, for he intended to have saved himself and his sight.

The Duke immediately disarmed himself and came to the King, showing him the closeness of his sight, and swore that he would never run against the King again. But if the King had been even a little hurt, the King's servants would have put the Duke in jeopardy. Then the King called his armourers and put all his pieces together and then took a spear and ran six courses very well, by which all men might perceive that he had no hurt, which was a great joy and comfort to all his subjects there present.

TREATMENT FROM THE TUDOR PERIOD

Though there appeared to be no lasting damage to His Majesty, his physicians would have still treated his head where the lance struck. Thomas Gale wrote in his chirurgeon handbook a treatment for head wounds that did not have damage to the cranium, or an injury to the head that did not crack or fracture the bone. While this book was written after his jousting accident, it is a good representation of what the chirurgeons could have done to treat Henry's head injury.

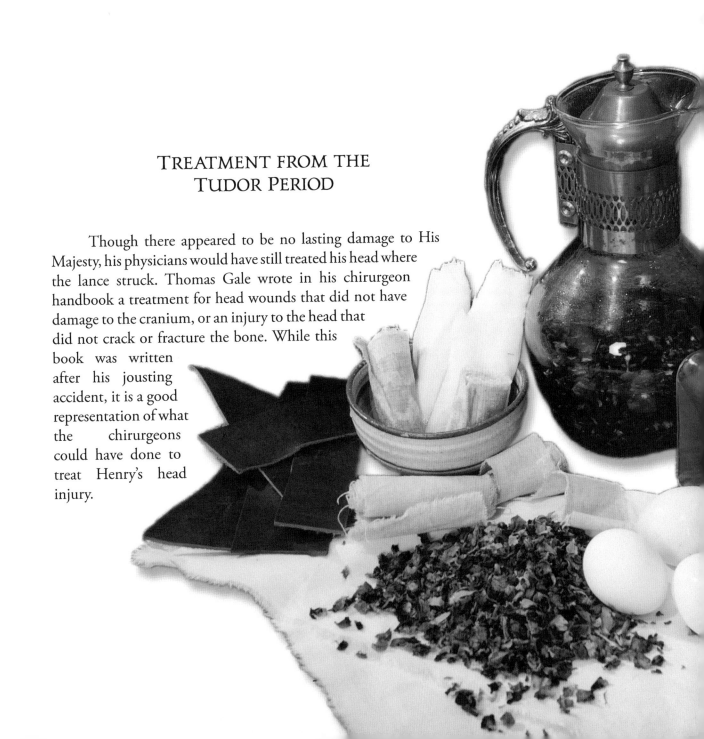

Head Injury Treatment
- Certaine Workes of Chirurgerie -
Thomas Gale

Thomas Gale wrote in his handbook of chirurgerie:

"

If the wounde be simple wythoute hurte of Cranium or losse of substance: then is the cure of it like the cure of other woundes to wiche, rolle, incarnate, and cicatrize. But yf the wounde be wyth the loss of substaunce then you must dyppe your tents and couer your plegeantes wyth incarnatyues, and Cicatrize the wounde with your accustomed pouders, unguents, emplasters, and other thyngs thereto belongynge. As touchynge stiching in the heade because manye speake agaynste it: I affyrme it to be not onelye profitable in small woundes, but also in great, most necessarye. For it kepeth the partes separated together, which rolling can not, it also causcth that the aire dothe not alter the part, which where if chaunceth it is verye hurtfull. And here I except great woundes in the fore parte of the heade whych maye not be stiched but on the syde. And putting in it oyle of roses which doth take awaye the payne of the neruous panicle inuestynge and couerynge Cranium, yf the wounde be so deepe and also it maketh the bones more easye to be taken oute, and taketh away the sharpenes of Mell when with it we intende to mundifie any inward panicle and defendeth from accidentes.

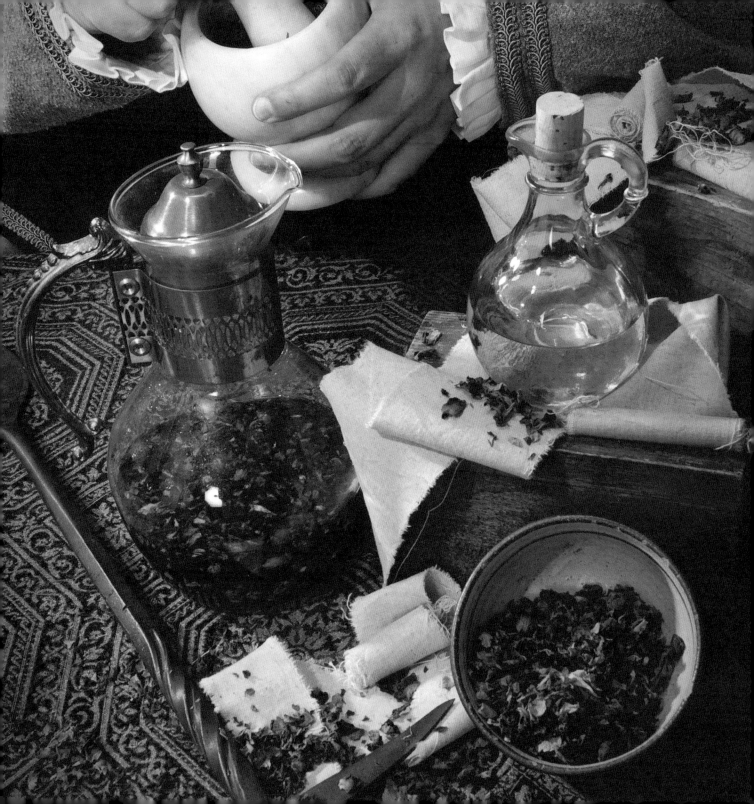

"If the wound be simple without hurt of cranium or loss of substance: then is the cure of it like the cure of other wounds to wash, roll, incarnate,[73] and cicatrize.[74] But if the wound be with the loss of substance then you must dip your tents and cover your plegeantes with incarnates, and cicatrize the wound with your accustomed powders, unguents,[75] plasters, and other things there to belonging. As touching stitching in the head because, any speak against it: I affirm it to be not only profitable in small wounds, but also in great, most necessary. For it keeps the parts separated together, which rolling cannot, it also causes that the air does not alter the part, which where if by chance it is very hurtful. And here I except great wounds in the fore part of the head which may not be stitched but on the side. And putting in it oil of roses which does take away the pain of the nervous panicle[76] investing and covering cranium, if the wound be so deep and also it makes the bones more the sharpness of mell[77] when with it we intend to mundify[78] any inward panicle and defend from accidents."

Rose oil was used to help to cleanse a wound to the head, helping to clean out particles and keeping it from becoming infected. Culpeper recorded how to make a compound oil: having bruised the herbs or flowers, place them into an earthen pot, and for every two or three handfuls of them, pour over a pint of oil. Cover the pot with paper, set it in the sun for about a fortnight or so, according to the heat of the sun. Then, having warmed it well by the fire, squeeze out the herb. To make the oil stronger, add more bruised herbs to the same oil and set in the sun as before. The more often you repeat this, the stronger the oil will be. Keep it in a stone or glass vessel for your use.[79] When recreating this treatment, I used olive oil because, according to Culpeper, olive oil did not hold any virtues but could take on the virtues of the herbs heated in it.

"Oil Olive, which is commonly known by the name of Salad Oil, I suppose because it is usually eaten with salads by them that love it; if it be pressed out of ripe olives, according to Galen, is temperate, and exceeds in no one quality."[80] Though *Complete Herbal* was published 1653, he references Galen's[81] thoughts on the virtues, or lack of virtues, of olive oil. This means that this treatment would have been focused on using the virtues of rose to treat the wound. John Gerard writes of the virtues of rose oil in *The Herbal or, General History of Plants*, "The oile doth mitigate all kindes of heat, and will not suffer inflammations or hot swellings to rise and being risen it doth at the first asswage[82] them."[83] The rose in this treatment was used based on the idea that it would be cooling, and keep the wound from causing the humours to get out of balance due to the heat of the inflammation.

Henry narrowly escaped a very serious injury; he could have received more than a cut to the head, he could have lost an eye, fractured his skull or died. He is also lucky that he escaped an infection. He also showed that at thirty-three he was not infallible and even a king can lose a joust now and again. In another three years, his beloved sport of tennis showed him that he was also vulnerable off the tilt field.

1527
TENNIS ACCIDENT

The jousting accident in 1527 was not the last time Henry was injured pursuing his love of athletics. Henry was an avid tennis player and was often upon the courts that his father had built at Richmond, Westminster, Windsor, Woodstock, and Wycombe, and the courts Henry VIII built at Hampton Court right after he was gifted the palace in 1528. Real tennis or the "game of kings" is different from the tennis that is seen at Wimbledon. The ancestor of the game of kings is likely to be *jeu de paume,* French for handball. It could have been played earlier, but it was at least played by the Romans and Greeks, and the Roman legionaries are thought to have brought the game north when they marched into Gaul. The game evolved through the middle ages. Courts had a length of 90 feet and a breadth of 30 feet. Players started to wear gloves to protect their hands and these gloves then ained gut strings. Eventually, a handle was added, making them similar to modern racquets.

"Though tennis is traditionally styled the Game of Kings early records show that it was the ecclesiastical high-ups who first put their stamp of approval on the game. Prelates, Abbots and minor clergy played it with almost religious fervour."[84] The first published rules of tennis were printed in 1592, in Paris, *Ordonnance du Royal et honourable Jeu de la Paulme.* The opening of the book says, "You gentlemen who desire to strive with another at tennis must play for the recreation of the body and the delectation of the mind, and must not indulge in swearing or in blasphemy against the name of God". In England, tennis truly was the game of kings. Henry was well-known for his prowess on the court. Sebastian Giustinian, Venetian Ambassador, wrote of Henry and his skill, "He is extremely fond of tennis, at which game it is the prettiest thing in the world to see him play, his fair skin glowing through a shirt of the finest texture."[85]

LETTERS FROM COURT

"By age thirty-six, Henry also suffered from a wrenched[86] foot in a tennis match causing him to don a black velvet slipper. This slipper, as it were, became a fashion statement throughout the court during 1527, the year of his injury. It is debatable whether the adoption of the slipper in English dress was due to the king's influence on fashion or was an attempt by his courtiers to show their sympathy for their injured king."[87] J. J. Scarisbrick, in his book *Henry VIII*, wrote this of the celebrations to do with the signing of the Treaty of Westminster. Henry was seen wearing a black slipper, and was recorded as sitting out the dances.[88] The treaty was signed on 30 April 1527, so if he was indeed sitting out of the celebrations due to his ankle we know that he wrenched his foot before 30 April.[89]

Most sources reference the tennis accident in 1527, however, there is a letter written on 20 March 1539, to Cardinal Wolsey, "Received your letters this morning, and went straight to Greenwich. As the King had wrenched his foot, could not see him till eleven, when I delivered him the letters which have tarried so long." It is not clear if he wrenched his foot twice or if there was an error in the year.

TREATMENTS FROM THE TUDOR PERIOD

I have included two treatments from *Certaine Workes of Chirurgerie*, by Thomas Gale, for Henry's wrenched ankle. One of the treatments is to stabilize the ankle, and the other to keep the humours in balance and keep the fluxes from causing the ankle to swell. Just like the treatment included for his first jousting accident was from Thomas Gale's book, both of these are from his book because the contents of his book are first-aid focused.

Wrenched Joint
- Certaine Workes of Chirurgerie -
Thomas Gale

"

When as the member luxated is brought in to his natural place you must wyth al diligence possible labour to confirme the part and kepe the member from slypping out again. Wherfore you shal anoint the place with oile of roses and then a fine and olde linen cloth wet also in oile of roses shalbe apllied to the member which bone you shall use stufes and clothes wet in the white of egges & lay them also on the ioynt. Last you shal wet your rollers in water and vinegar mixed together and rol the member therwith. And if necessitie doth require you maye furthermore make splents of lether or pasted paper and apply them about the ioynt. But give diligence lest the part be too strait bound and rolled for feare of inflammation. These thinges thus finished laye the member in his natural figure & shape. Neyther shal you (exept fome great and ill accident happen) lose the roller & open the member, before the vij, or tenth day at the lest. Auicenna willeth that in the case you shall not use hote clothes or medicines for fear of fluxe and inflammation but rather some refrigeratiue cerote.

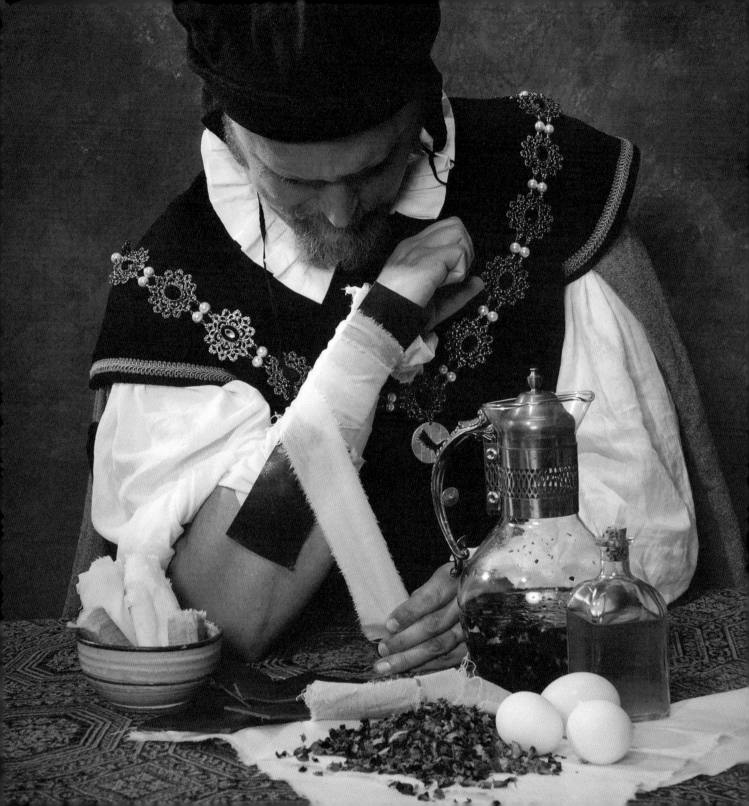

"When as the member luxated[91] is brought in to his natural place you must with all diligence possible, labour to confirm the part and keep the member from slipping out again. Wherefore you shall anoint the place with oil of roses and then a fine and old linen cloth, wet also in oil of roses, shall be applied to the member which bone you shall use stuff and clothes wet in the white of eggs and lay them also on the joint. Last you shall wet your rollers[92] in water and vinegar mixed together and roll the member therewith. And if necessity does require you may furthermore make splints of leather or pasted paper and apply them about the joint. But give diligence lest the part be too strait bound and rolled for fear of inflammation. These things thus finished lay the member in his natural figure and shape. Neither shall you (except from great and ill accident happen) lose the roller and open the member, before the seventh, or tenth day at the least. Avicenna[93] wills that in the case you shall not use hot clothes or medicines for fear of flux and inflammation but rather some refrigerative cerate."[94]

Based on this passage the first thing to do is to bring the joint back to its natural position, then you must with all thoroughness keep the joint from moving again. Then you should anoint the joint with oil of roses and then a fine and old linen cloth, also soaked with oil of roses, shall be applied to the member. Then apply cloths dampened with egg whites to the joint. Lastly, you should wet your rollers in water and vinegar mixed together and roll them on the joint. If needed, you could also make splints of leather or pasted paper and apply them to the joint. But be careful, for if the part is too tightly bound and rolled then the joint could flux or become inflamed.

CERTAINE VVORKES

of Chirurgerie, nevvly compiled and
published by Thomas Gale, Master in Chirurgerie.

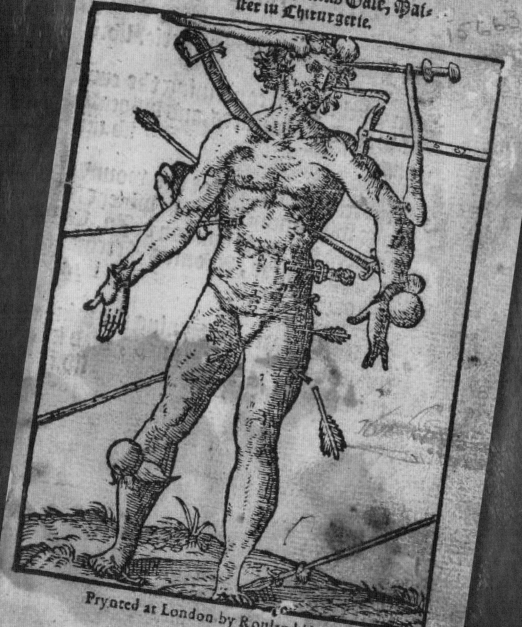

Prynted at London by Rouland Hall.

To Balance the Humours
- Certaine Workes of Chirurgerie -
Thomas Gale

"

The member luxated being reduced to hys natural place and confirmed in the same, & also hauing his perfit shape & figure: there remaineth to defend the same from ill accidentes, or if such happen or thou be called to the cure to put them away. In the defending the member you shal labour to kepe the member from flux of humours for if there be a flux, then shal there folow both Dolour and inflammation. Therfore strengthen the member with apt & conuenient, medicines set out in diuers parts of the worke. Also let him use thin and smal diet, purgien, and letting blood: for these so meruailously auert the flux from the affected member. But if it chance that there is already accidentes or thou come to the pacient, as dolour or inflammation, then thou shalt not out the member luxated into the place before thou haste cured the accidentes. Therefore these things sufficientlye declared as much as the nature of an Enchiridion requireth touching the methodicall curinge of woundes both in similer and instrumentall members, also of fractures & dislocations I will speake brefely & taken of members and then seace my penne for this present.[85]

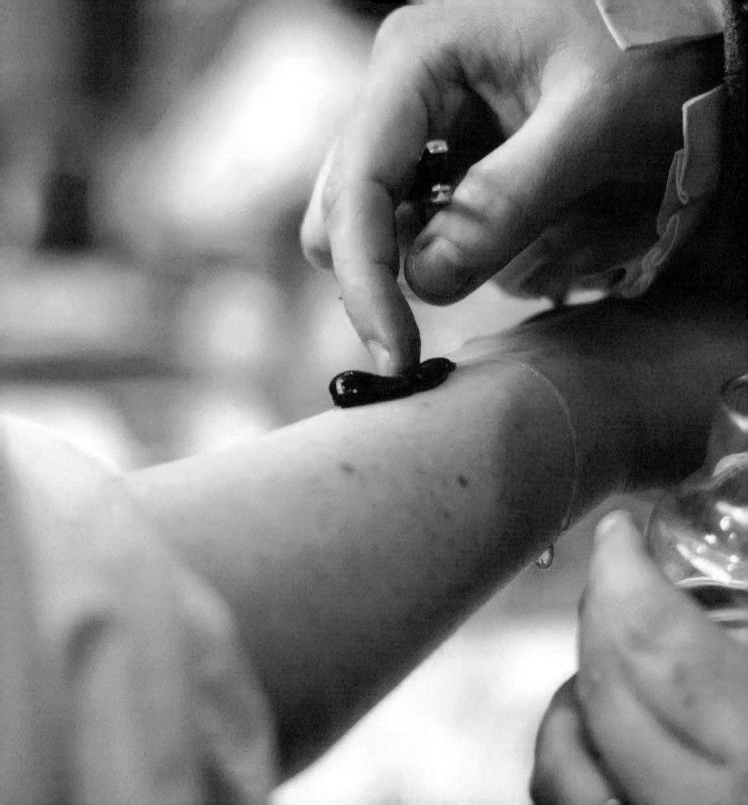

"The member luxated being reduced to his natural place and confirmed in the same, and also having his perfect shape and figure: there remains to defend the same from ill accidents, or if such happen or thou be called to the cure to put them away. In the defending the member you shall labour to keep the member from flux of humours for if there be a flux, then shall there follow both dolour[96] and inflammation. Therefore, strengthen the member with apt and convenient, medicines set out in divers[97] parts of the work. Also let him use thin and small diet, purging, and letting blood: for these so marvellously avert the flux from the affected member. But if it chances that there are already accidents or thou come to the patient, as dolour or inflammation, then thou shalt not put the member luxated into the place before thou hast cured the accidents. Therefore, these things sufficiently declared as much as the nature of an enchiridion[98] requires touching the methodical curing of wounds both in similar and instrumental members, also of fractures and dislocations I will speak briefly and taken of members and then cease my pen for this present."

To keep the fluxes from causing the joint to swell, Gale wrote that the patient should eat a small diet, purge, and a physician should perform blood-letting. Though translated from Arabic to Latin between 100 and 200 years before Henry was born, very few medical books cover the diet of the sick like the *Tacuinum Sanitatis*, focusing largely on the correct food to help keep or rebalance the humours of the body. Four versions were found across Europe, and it gives a wonderful look into the theory of food affecting the humours of the body, as well as the correct air and activates needed to affect the humours. For example, it says that rye can be used to "break down the concentration of humours."

Purging is the second way he suggested to help the flow of fluxes, and it was a common treatment. Within Dioscorides' *De Materia Medica*, there are 112 treatments to purge the body, including old wine with honey, seawater, and a wine made with scammony.

The third way to balance the humours is through blood-letting, and it is separated into a generalized method done by venesection[99] and arteriotomy,[100] and a controlled technique done by scarification,[101] with cupping and leeches. In the photograph, is my medical leech photographed by Heather Morgan-Leist during a presentation at a historical recreation event. Another way to bleed a patient was with a fleam. The fleam was used to make small holes, limiting the amount of blood released. It is likely that a careful royal physician would use this method, or possibly leeches, as opposed to cutting or methods that would take large amounts of blood.

Henry's trouble with his ankle would not be the last issue with his legs that he would face, and was one of the milder issues he had. His esteemed legs would become a curse.

1527/28
SWOLLEN LEGS AND
ULCERATED LEFT LEG

Henry's legs began to swell, and were troubled with varicose veins, and he developed an ulcer on his left thigh. It is most plausible that much of the trouble with his legs was due to poor circulation caused by the tight garters he wore to show off the calves of which he was so proud. His calves were so often the talk of the court.[102]

Swollen legs and varicose veins can lead to ulcers, or another opinion is that the ulcers were from osteomyelitis[103] due to tiny fractures in the femur bone from jarring the bones in activities like jousting.[104] Sir Arthur Salusbury MacNalty writes that one of Henry VIII's progresses was held up in Canterbury in 1527 due to his "sorre leg." This was treated by Thomas Vicary, a royal serjeant-surgeon.[105]

TREATMENTS FROM THE TUDOR PERIOD

There are quite a few treatments for legs and swelling in the medical texts from Henry's physicians. I have included one treatment for swollen legs taken from *Certain works of Chirurgerie*, a treatment for pain from the *Prescription Book of Henry VIII*, and a poultice taken from Bullein's work to treat the ulcer.

THYS PLASTER WAS DEVISED FOR KING HENRIE THE EYGHTE TO AMENDE THE SWELLYNG IN HIS LEGGES - CERTAINE WORKES OF CHIRURGERIE- THOMAS GALE

Take the rotes of Marche Malowes washe & picke them cleane, then slitte them and take oute the inner pithe and caste it away, and take the upper fayre whyte parte and cut them in smalle peeces, and brouse then in a morter and thereof take one pounde and putte them in a newe earthen pote and add therto of lynesede and fenegreeke ana. two onces a litle brosed in a morter, then put thereto malmsie and whyte wyne ana. a pynte, and sturre altogether and lette them stande infused, two or three dayes, then set them ouer a soft fire and sturre it well tyll it waxe thycke and slimme, then take it of and straine it through newe canues clothe, and thus haue your mucylage readye and then to make your plaster. Take fyne Oyle of Roses a quarte and washe it will wyth whyte wyne and rose water. Then take the oyle cleane from the water and wyne, & set it over the fire in a brase pan always sturringe it and put thereto the pouder of

cont.

whyte wyne and rose water. Then take
...le cleane from the water and wyne, & set
...er the fire in a brase pan alwaies sturrings
...d put thereto the pouder of.

Lythargyri auri	} ana, viij. vnces.
Lythargyri argenti,	
Cerusæ,	vi. vnces.
Corallo. rub.	ij. vnces.
Boli armoniaci	} ana one vnce.
Sangui. draconis,	

And in anye wyse make them in fyne pouder
...arsid, then put them into the oyle ouer the fire
...lwaies styring, and let not the fier be to bigge
...o2 burning of the stuffe, and when it beginneth
...to waxe thicke, then put in of the sayd mucylage
...x. vnces by litle and little at ones, o2 els it wyll
boile ouer the pan, and when it is boiled enough
ye shall perceyue by the hardnes o2 softnes therof, if thou d2ope a lytle of it on a dishe botome o2
cold stone then take it from the fy2e, and whē it
is nere cold, make it in roules and lape them in
parchment, and kepe them to your vse.

Emplastrum pro Chameleontiasi nostræ
inuentionis.

Rec.

Lythargyri auri	} Ana, viij. vnces
Lythargyri argenti,	
Cerusae	vi. vnces.
Corallo. rub	ij. vnces.
Boli armoniaci.	
Sangui. Draconis,	} Ana one vnce.

And in anye wyse make them in fyne pouder
searsid, then put them into the oyle ouer
the fire alwaies styring, and let not the fier
be to bigge for burning of the stuffe, and
when it beginneth to waxe thicke, then put
in of the sayd mucylage x unces by litle
and little at ones, or els it wyll boile ouer
the pan, and when it is boiled enough ye
shall perceyue by the hardnes or softness
therof, if thou drope a lytle of it on a
dishe botome or cold stone then take
it from the fyre, and when it is nere
cold, make it in roules and lape them in
parchment, and kepe them to you use. [106]

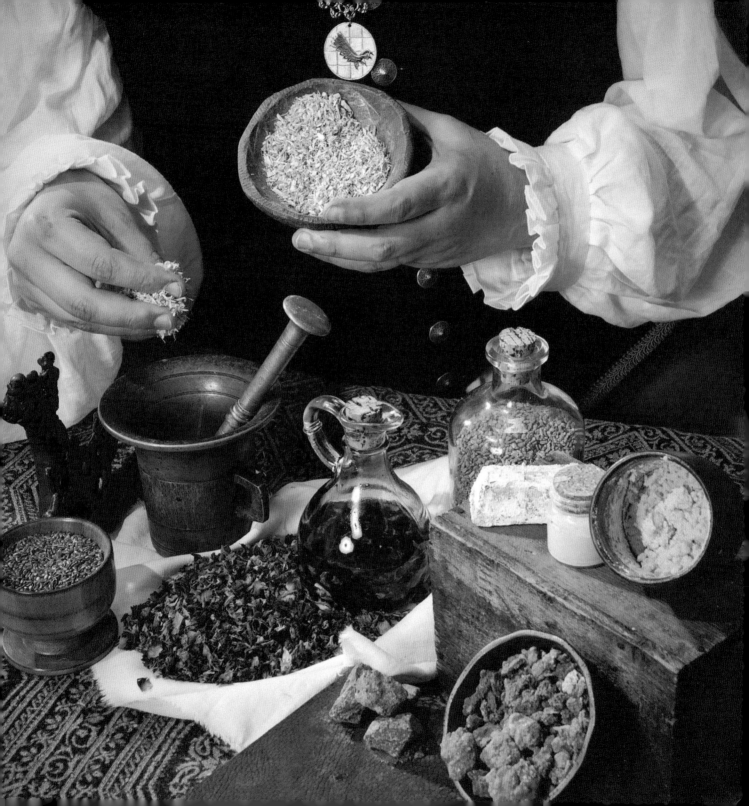

"Take the roots of marshmallow, wash & pick them clean, then cut them and take out the inner pith and cast it away, and take the upper fair white part and cut them in small pieces, and bruise them in a mortar and thereof take one pound and put them in a new earthen pot and add thereto of linseed and fenugreek, two ounces, a little bruised in a mortar, then put thereto malmsey and white wine, one pint, and stir altogether and let them stand infused, two or three days, then set them over a soft fire and stir it well, till it wax[107] thick and slim,[108] then take it off and strain through new canvas cloth, and thus have your mucilage[109] ready and then to make your plaster. Take fine oil of roses, a quart, and wash it well with white wine and rose water. Then take the oil clean from the water and wine, and set it over the fire in a brass pan always stirring it and put thereto the powder of

Gold-Lead	}	8 ounces
Silver Lead		
Ceruse		6 ounces
Red Coral		2 ounces
Lump ammoniacum	}	1 ounces.
Dragon's Blood		

And in any wise make them in fine powder searsed, then put them into the oil over the fire always stirring, and let not the fire be too big for burning of the stuff, and when it begins to wax thick, then put in of the said mucilage ten ounces by little and little at once, or else it will boil over the pan, and when it is boiled enough you shall perceive by the hardness or softness thereof, if thou drop a little of it on a dish bottom or cold stone then take it from the fire, and when it is near cold, make it in rolls and lap[110] them in parchment, and keep them for your use."

Thomas Gale writes the above passage about a plaster made for Henry's swollen legs. He says to prepare marshmallow root,[111] and add two ounces each of linseed and fenugreek, both ground, and then add a pint each of malmsey (a strong, sweet wine imported from Greece and the eastern Mediterranean islands) and white wine. Mix them and then let stand for two to three days, then place over a low fire and stir it well, until it is thick. Then take it off and strain, and you have your mucilage. Set this aside and prepare the other ingredients for the plaster. Take a quart of rose oil, and wash it well with white wine and rose water. Put the oil over a fire and continue to stir it as you add eight ounces of gold lead (now called lead-tin yellow) and silver lead (known as white lead). Also add six ounces of the white lead and vinegar-based make-up cream called ceruse, two ounces of a red coral, and one ounce each of lump ammoniacum[112] and dragon's blood.[113] Keep the fire medium hot, not too hot or too cold, and when it begins to thicken, put in ten ounces of the mucilage, that was previously set aside, little by little, or it could boil over. When it is boiled enough and cooled a little, make it into rolls and wrap in parchment; keep for use.

The parts of this treatment that should be mentioned, as they are more harmful than they can be helpful, are the three types of lead used: ceruse, gold lead, and silver lead. It is astounding to the modern mind to think of rubbing on the skin a treatment that contains three types of lead. The neurological side-effects of lead are well-known, but some of the other physical effects on the body include toxic stress on the kidneys, inhibited production of red blood cells, abdominal pain, high blood pressure, and fertility issues.[114] Today, we know these side effects, but back then, and going as far back as the 1st century, it was thought that lead was beneficial. Dioscorides wrote that lead salts like gold and silver lead are "most effectively mixed with gentle plasters called lipara, and is effective with plasters that are not corrosive — promoting the growth of flesh in a wound or sore, and forming new skin."[115]

PAIN TREATMENT
- HENRY'S PRESCRIPTION BOOK -
HENRY VIII AND HIS PHYSICIANS

"

The King Majesty's Plaster made at westmor to mitigate payne

Take a pynt of rose water, and half a pynt of white wyne, and boyle threw these thinges following of violett leaves, chamomile floweres, peressemyn flowers, borage flowers of the wall fellw flowers of the sede of prvett an Z 1. Fyll the one half be consumed the ...[illegible, damaged] and wt this decoction drawe the mucellage of juyuses of the soedes of holyocke of ...[illegible, damaged], and of reysynes - an Z 2. Then take oyle of rosyes viij unces, and oyle of white lyllyes iij Z well washed in warme white wyne iiij or v tymes. Drain the wyne from thr oyle and putt therto finly pouldered and perparaded of lytherge of golde leade iiij vnces of redde corall Z ij rasure eborio Z j of jacincte di[m] unce, of margarite di[m] unce, boyle these poulders and your oyle to gether over a soft fyre evermore stiring and feding it in your mucilage by lytle and lytle tyll it be plaster lyke, and ...[illegible] st of all in the coolying putt in fynly pouldered chamomill flowers of violett flowers of borage flowers an Z j of that emplastum[116]

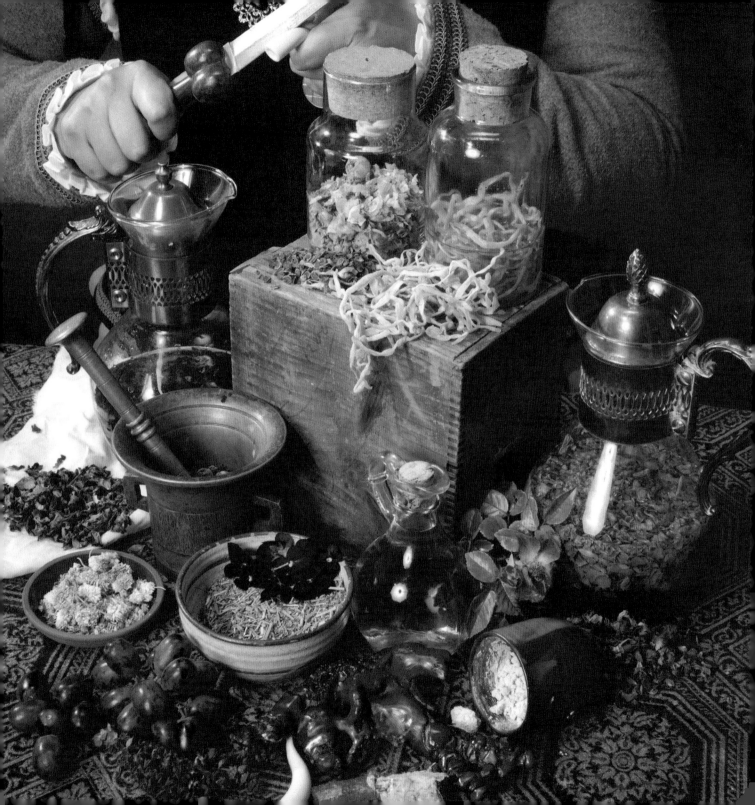

"The King Majesty's Plaster made at Westmorland to mitigate pain.

Take a pint of rose water, and half a pint of white wine, and boil through these things following of violet leaves, chamomile flowers, persimmon flowers, borage flowers of the wall, fellwort flowers of the seed of privet a dram 1. Fill the one half be consumed the [illegible] and with this decoction draw the mucilage of juices. Of the seeds of hollyhocks of [illegible], and of raisins – an 2 drams. Then take oil of roses, 8 ounces, and oil of white lilies 3 drams well washed in warm white wine 4 or 5 times. Drain the wine from the oil and put thereto finely powdered and prepared of litharge of gold lead 4 ounces, of red coral 2 dram, shaved ivory 1 dram, of jacinth 1/2 ounce, of marguerite 1/2 ounce, boil these powders and your oil together over a soft fire evermore stirring and feeding it in your mucilage by little and little till it be plaster like, and [illegible]st of all in the cooling put in finely powdered chamomile flowers of violet flowers of borage flowers 1 dram, of that emplastum"

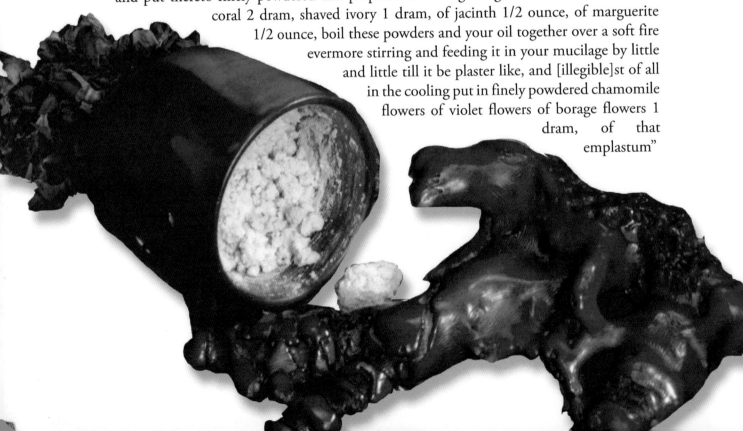

It is possible that this treatment was just titled as "His King Majesty's" to make it seem more important or reliable, however, it was in his physician's prescription book, and is likely to have actually been used to treat Henry, or it could have even been made by Henry, as he was an amateur apothecary. To make the treatment, take violet leaves, chamomile flowers, persimmon[117] flowers, borage flowers, fellwort[118] herb, and privet seed, from the genus *Ligustrum*. Add these to white wine and rose water, and boil. After one-half of the fluid has been boiled off, drain the juices off to get the mucilage, and set aside. Wash oil of roses and lily with warm white wine and then add hollyhock seed, raisins, and finely powdered gold lead, red coral, shaved ivory, jacinth, and marguerite. Jacinth could be one of two ingredients, an orange-red stone or a purple or blue flower modernly called hyacinth. However, as jacinth is in the recipe sandwiched between ivory and marguerite, a mica like stone, it is not the flower, but the mineral that the physicians are referring to. Boil this mixture and add the mucilage slowly until it is plaster-like. After it has cooled, put in finely powdered chamomile flowers, violet flowers and borage flower.

There are no studies that show the effectiveness of borage flower on pain, other than a possible use for rheumatoid arthritis, but the plant contains gamma-linolenic acid which may be an anti-inflammatory and it is used modernly as an astringent.[119] Violets are used for some skin conditions by herbalists today, but it seems to have no uses for pain. Chamomile flowers contain alpha-bisabolol, however, and studies have shown it could help wounds to heal,[120] and while this may not directly help with pain, a healed wound of course is less painful.

ULCER TREATMENT
- BULLEIN'S BULWARKE OF DEFENCE -
WILLIAM BULLEIN

"

MYROBALANVM is a noble fruicte of Inde lyke Plumbes whych hath vertue to purge superfluous humours, and comforteth nature, and who so vseth to eate often of Myrobalans being condite, shall not seeme olde, sayth Mesue, and maketh pure couler. There bee .5. kindes of theym, as Flauj, Chepuli, Indicj. or Nigrj, Empelicj, and Belliricj, which do differ one from the other: for ý Flauj, and Chepulj, do grow both vpon one tree, for the Flauj are gathered vnripe, and the Chepulj haue their full nature and rypenesse. Myrobalans, Flauj, Indicj, Chepulj, and Belliricj, be colde in the first, and dry in the second degree Empelicj are colde and dry in the first degree, and be good for the Lyuer, Gaule, Splene, Raynes, and Bladder: and put in infusion of the Iuyce of Quinces, standing .24. houres, and then strayned, then put prepared Scammonie, they wil purge choller, as for example: Take Myrobalans Flauj. ʒ.j. the iuyce or syrupe simple of Quinces. ʒ.iiij. stampe your Myrobalans, and then mingle them wyth the sayd Iuyce, the Iuyce being made warme, and let it stand in a close stone vessell .24. houres, then strayne it forth, whan this is done, beate your prepared Scammonie fine into pouder. ʒ.iiij. and temper it together, putting it in a close warme place to dry it by little & little, and of thys ʒ.j. or litle more wil purge choller, & humours superfluous without hurte. Myrobalans may be stamped with the Syrup of Wormewoode, & then sodden with ý infusion of Agarike, & Rhabarbe, to purge flegme & choller: it may be drawen with Chassia & Manna, for noble persons or People of tender nature. This fruict defendeth the body from corruption, trimbling of the heart, heauines, Melancholy, & bringeth to nature, Cleanlynesse, fauour, & myrth. And drawen wyth Fentil water and Sugar, it wyl clense the sight to bee dropped into them morning and euening. The pouder of them wyth Rosen wyll heale sore Ulcers.[121]

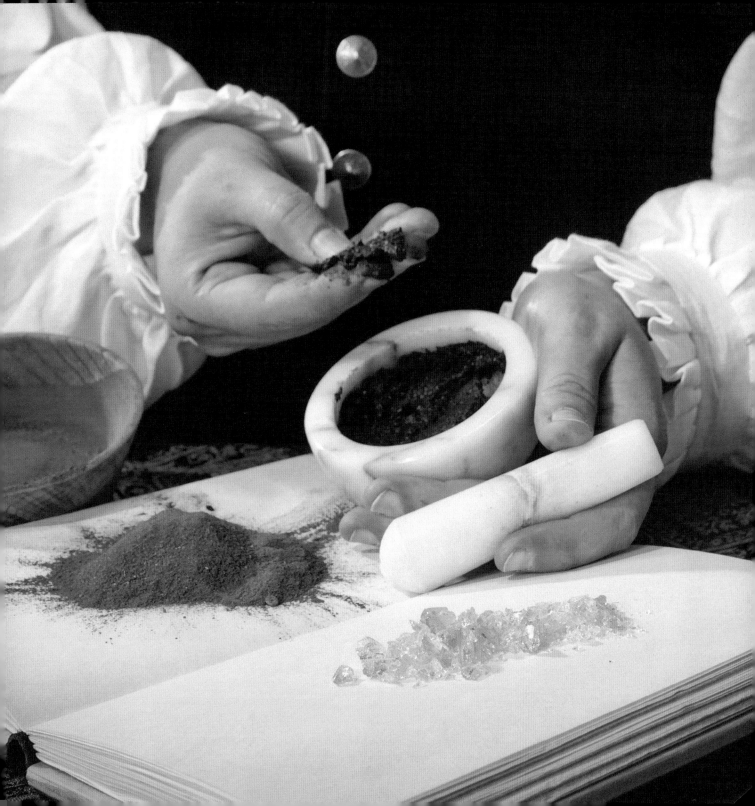

"Myrobalan is a noble fruit of India like plums which has virtues to purge superfluous humours, and comforting nature and whoso used to eat often of myrobalans being condite, shall not seem old, sayeth Mesue,[122] and makes pure colour. There be five kinds of them, as *flaui*, *chepuli*, *indici* or *nigri*, *empelici*, and *bellirici*, which do differ one from the other: for *flaui*, and *chepuli*, do grow both upon one tree, for the *flaui* are gathered unripe, and the *chepuli* have their full nature and ripeness. Myrobalans, *flaui*, *indici*, *chepuli*, and *bellirici*, be cold in the first, and dry in the second degree *empelici* are cold and dry in the first degree, and be good for the liver, gall, spleen, kidneys, and bladder: and put in infusion of the juice of quinces, standing 24 hours, and then strained, then put prepared scammony,[123] they will purge choler, as for example: take myrobalans *flaui* one ounce, the juice or syrup simple of quinces four ounces, stamp your myrobalans, and then mingle them with the said juice, the juice being made warm, and let it stand in a closed stone vessel 24 hours, then strain it forth, when this is done, beat your prepared scammony fine into powder 4 ounces, and temper it together, putting it in a closed warm place to dry it by little and little, and of this one dram or little more will purge choler, and humours superfluous without hurt. Myrobalans may be stamped with the syrup of wormwood, and then sodden with the infusion of agaric, and rhubarb, to purge phlegm and choler: it may be drawn with cassia & manna, for noble persons or people of tender nature. This fruit defends the body from corruption, trembling of the heart, heaviness, melancholy, and brings to nature, cleanliness, favour, and mirth. And drawn with [fentil] water and sugar, it will cleanse the sight to be dropped into them morning and evening. The powder of them with rosin will heal sore ulcers."

Dioscorides writes about both myrobalan and a wine made with rosin. "Myrobalan is the fruit of a tree like myrica, similar to hazelnut. That within is pressed like bitter almonds, and it yields a liquid that they use for precious ointments instead of oil. It grows in Ethiopia, Egypt, Arabia, and in Petra, a town in Judaea. That which is new, full, white, and easily peeled is the best. This, pounded into small pieces and a teaspoonful taken in a drink with posca reduces the spleen, and it is also laid on it with oat meal. It is used with honey and water on gout. Boiled with vinegar it raises out scabies and leprosy. It is used with saltpeter for leprosy and black scars. With urine it takes away freckles, varicose veins, sunburn, and pustules on the face. With honey water it induces vomiting, and loosens the intestines, but is very bad for the stomach. The oil (taken as a drink) is astringent to the bowels…"[124]

Bullein wrote in his herbal of a treatment made from the powder of myrobalan. Mixing the powder of myrobalan with rosin will heal sore ulcers when applied topically as a plaster. Rosin is a solid amber-coloured residue obtained after the distillation of crude turpentine extracted from pine stumps. Bullein writes that there are five types of myrobalan. I used black myrobalan, a medium to large deciduous tree, which can also be used as a fibre dye. *Terminalia chebula* is black myrobalan's botanical name and is related to approximately 100 species of flowering trees, including a handful of almond trees.

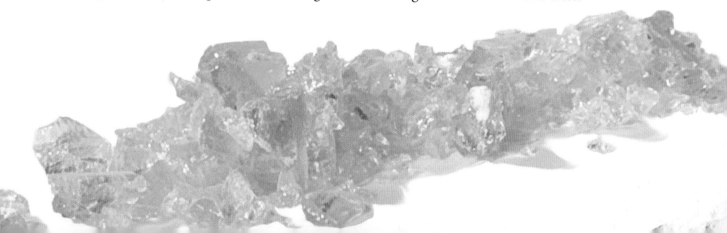

1536
SECOND JOUSTING ACCIDENT

The idea of jousting has been credited to Godfrey de Preuilly, a Frenchman. Godfrey wrote the rules in 1066, the same year that the Normans conquered the English at the Battle of Hastings. Jousting is a potentially dangerous activity and it is said that Godfrey died in the first ever tournament.

Jousting tournaments were entertainments devised by rich nobles to enable knights to practise their martial skills. They participated in mock battles or single combat jousting, as well as events on horseback. This practice continued for centuries, despite the deaths and serious injuries which sometimes happened.

In 1536, the last year of Anne Boleyn's life, Anne was pregnant again. The royal couple were hoping for the boy that Henry desired so much. Sadly, for Anne, it was not to be. Henry, while jousting at Greenwich, had the second jousting accident of his life. It is said that the King was unseated from his horse and crashed to the ground with the fully-armoured horse landing on top of him. He remained unconscious ('without speech') for two hours. His legs were crushed in the fall and he may have sustained fractures. There was such concern over the potential severity of his injuries that the queen is said to have miscarried shortly after hearing of the accident.[125]

LETTERS FROM COURT

On 29 January, Chapuys wrote to Charles V, "On the day of the interment the Concubine had an abortion which seemed to be a male child which she had not borne 3½ months, at which the King has shown great distress. The said concubine wished to lay the blame on the Duke of Norfolk, whom she hates, saying he frightened her by bringing the news of the fall the King had six days before." The same day, Chapuys wrote to Granvelle, "On the eve of the Conversion of St. Paul, the King being mounted on a great horse to run at the lists, both fell so heavily that everyone thought it a miracle he was not killed, but he sustained no injury. Thinks he might ask of fortune for what greater misfortune he is reserved, like the other tyrant who escaped from the fall of the horse, in which all the rest were smothered, and soon after died."[126]

On 12 February, shortly after the accident, the Bishop of Faenza wrote to the Prothonotary Ambrogio, "Hear that the king of England has had a fall from his horse, and was thought to be dead for two hours. His lady miscarried in consequence."[127]

TREATMENTS FROM THE TUDOR PERIOD

The force of the horse landing on Henry's legs was likely to have done much internal damage, but it appears from the sources at the time that there was not much damage done to the outside of his legs. To treat wounds that are "deep and hidden wounds which cannot be well perceived," I have included two treatments from *Certain Works of Chirurgerie* by Thomas Gale, located in *The First Book of the Enchiridion*, one a wound flush and the other a healing plaster.

WOUND FLUSH
- CERTAINE WORKES OF CHIRURGERIE -
THOMAS GALE

"

In this kind of woundes the cure is done two sundry ways. First if the place may suffer it without hurt of vaines, arteries, & nerues, is to delate the wounde with tentes of gentian or of a sponge and after make it open & large wyth insicion. The other is if the first waye cannot be done without daunger, to put into the wounde a probe or waxe candle, until you come to the end of the wounde, and make there an yssue that by this way the matter in the wound may be clensed with some mendificatiue lotion conuaied in to the wound by a syring. Let your rolling also be such ý it be lose at the orifie of your wound, for otherwise you shal kepe ý matter stil in ý wound. Neither shall you in mundifiynge the wounde thurst out the mater, for so doing you shal thurst out the indigest matter in colour of blood & hinder much the cure of the wounde. As Brunswik maketh mention of a certayne barbour who had no knowledge in Chirurgery, and yet wold take upon him to practise. Thys Barbour (hauing a pacient wounded in the arme) did every day thurst out so much bloude and brought such accidentes to the parte, that yf Brunswyke had not fortunatly come, the barbours pacient had loste hys arme. Suche is the fruictes of blynde Emperikes. You shall also aboue the wounde applye some defensiue, and on the wound some mundificatiue, and make your iniections wyth a syring untill the water come forth of the same colour it was put in. the water bled for iniections is made in this maner.

Rec. Mellis rosacei.	vj.vnces:
Rosarum rubearum. Florum camomilli.	} Ana iij ounce.
Mastiches. Ireos.	} Ana j. ounce
Thuris	halfe a vnce.
Mirrhae.	i.dragme
Vini albi.	ij.pound.
Aquarú plantaginis vtriusqȝ. Rosarum. Caprifolij. Foliorum quercus.[128]	} Ana, a pound.

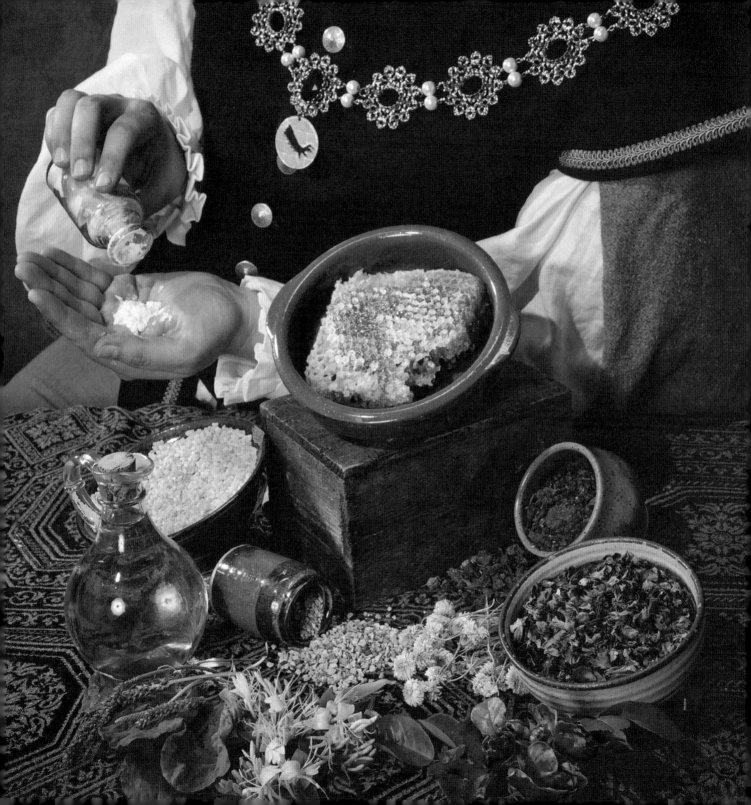

"In these kinds of wounds the cure is done two sundry ways. First if the place may suffer it without hurt of veins, arteries, and nerves, is to dilate the wound with tentes of gentian[129] or of a sponge and after make it open and large with incision. The other is if the first way cannot be done without danger, to put into the wound a probe or wax candle, until you come to the end of the wound, and make there an issue that by this way the matter in to the wound may be cleansed with some mundificative[130] lotion conveyed in the wound by a syringe. Let your rolling[131] also be such that it be loose at the orifice of your wound, for otherwise you shall keep the matter still in the wound. Neither shall you in mundiving the wound thrust out the matter, for so doing you shall thrust out the indigest[132] matter in colour of blood & hinder much the cure of the wound. As Brunswick makes mention of a certain barber who had no knowledge in Chirurgery, and yet would take upon him to practise. This Barber (having a patient wounded in the arm) did every day draw out so much blood and brought such accidents to the part, that if Brunswick had not fortunately come, the barber's patient [would have] lost his arm. Such is the fruits of blind empirics. You shall also above the wound apply some defensive, and on the wound, some mundificative, and make your injections with a syringe until the water come forth of the same colour it was put in. The water bled for injections is made in this manner.

Rose Honey	6 ounces
Red Rose Leaves	
Chamomile Blossoms	} 3 ounces
Mastic Gum[133]	
Orris[134]	} 1 ounce
Frankincense	half an ounce
Myrrh	1 dram
White wine	2 pounds
Plantain water from both species[135]	
Rose	
Honeysuckle	} 1 pound
Oak blossoms	

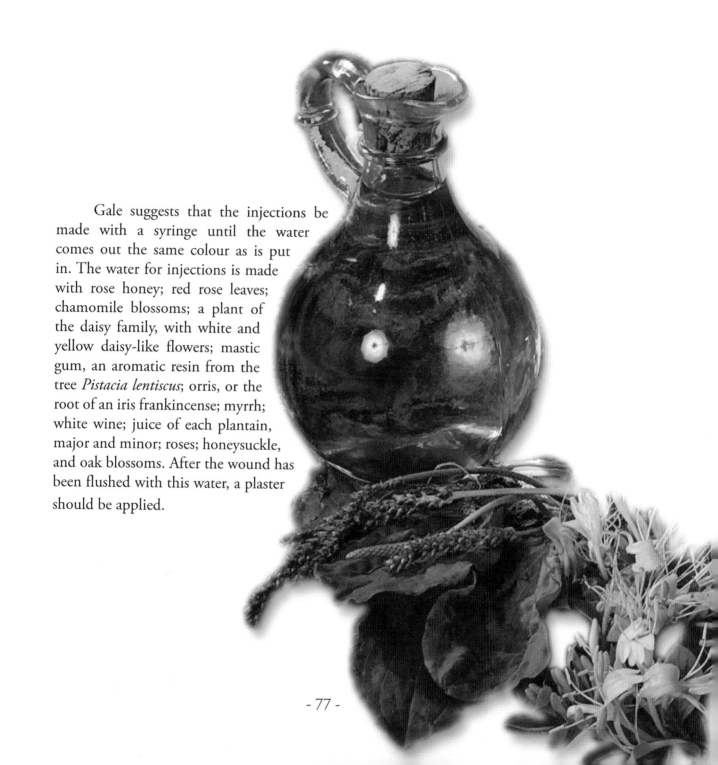

Gale suggests that the injections be made with a syringe until the water comes out the same colour as is put in. The water for injections is made with rose honey; red rose leaves; chamomile blossoms; a plant of the daisy family, with white and yellow daisy-like flowers; mastic gum, an aromatic resin from the tree *Pistacia lentiscus*; orris, or the root of an iris frankincense; myrrh; white wine; juice of each plantain, major and minor; roses; honeysuckle, and oak blossoms. After the wound has been flushed with this water, a plaster should be applied.

Wound Cleansing Plaster
- Certaine Workes of Chirurgerie -
Thomas Gale

A mundicatiue
Vnguenti egyptiaci.   ij. Vnces.
Aluminis   i vnce
Olibani   halfe a vnce
Mirrhae.   j.dragme
Vini rubei   tvvo pound,bulliant pulliant[136]

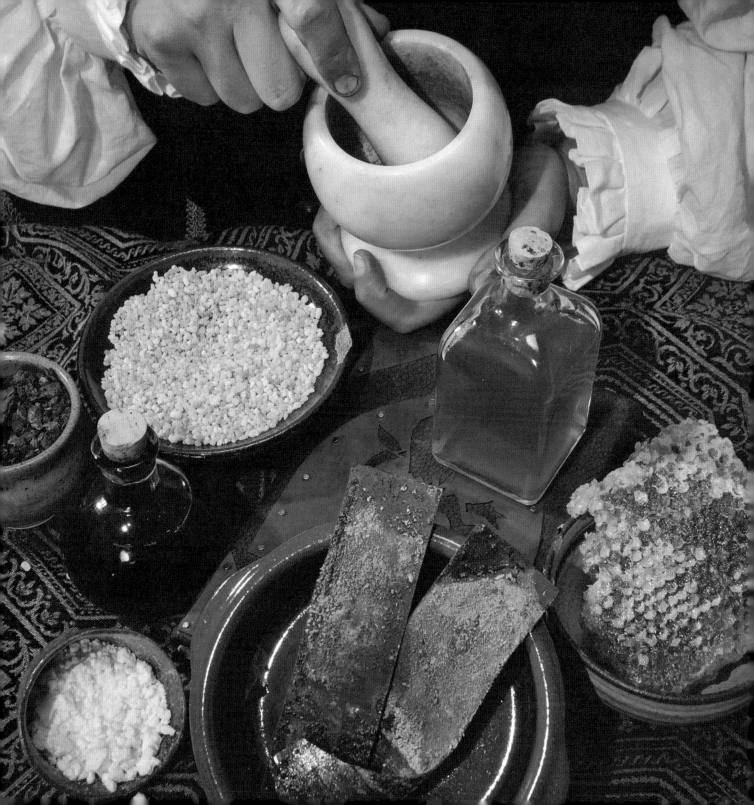

"A mundicative

Egyptian ointment[137]	2 ounces
Alum[138]	1 ounce
Frankincense	1/2 ounce
Myrrh	1 dram
Red Wine	2 pounds boil"

The mundificative to be applied to the wound is made with two ounces of Egyptian ointment, alum, frankincense and myrrh, boiled in red wine. Culpeper wrote that the Greeks' emplaisters consisted of these ingredients, metals, stones, diverse sorts of earth, faeces, juices, liquors, seeds, roots, herbs, excrements of creatures, wax, rosin, or gums.[139] This differs from a poultice, made from just plant material, because of the alum and the Egyptian ointment. Verdigris, one of the three ingredients in the *aegyptiacum* unguent, is made with copper, and alum is an aluminium salt, therefore making this a plaster and not a poultice.

The year 1536 not only saw the miscarriage of Anne Boleyn's last child and her own death by the sword of an executioner on 19 May, it saw the rise of the next queen of England. Jane Seymour became betrothed to Henry VIII on 20 May. While the beginning of the year was filled with sorrow, there was hope that as the year ended Henry's life would start to improve. It was not long, however, before he faced another serious health issue.

1537
ULCERATED LEGS

January of 1537 saw a rebellion in Cumberland and Westmorland led by Sir Francis Bigod. The Bigod rebellion was a rebellion by English Roman Catholics because they felt that Henry was not keeping the promises he made after the Pilgrimage of Grace,[140] the year before. Francis Bigod and his company were shortly arrested. The rebellion, and specifically the trial, was recorded in *Letters and Papers*: "Constable, Bigod, &c., are brought up and plead not guilty. Entry of the return of the jury, who are sworn and charged and retire to consider their verdict. Before they return Percy, Sir John Bulmer, Cheyne, and Hamerton plead guilty. The jury return and find Constable, Bigod, Lumley, and Aske guilty; as to Percy, Bulmer, Cheyne, and Hamerton (their plea of guilty being recorded) the jury are exonerated from giving any verdict. As to Ralph Bulmer they are with the assent of the court and of the King's serjeants-at-law and attorney exonerated from giving any verdict. The King's serjeants and attorney pray judgment."[141]

Ultimately, Sir Francis Bigod was hanged at Tyburn. Thomas Darcy, 1st Baron Darcy of Darcy, and Lord John Husee were both beheaded. Thomas Moigne, who had been elected Member of Parliament for Lincolnshire, was hanged, drawn and quartered. Sir Robert Constable and Robert Aske were both hanged in chains. Sir Nicholas Tempest, Bowbearer of the Forest of Bowland, was hanged at Tyburn. Sir John Bulmer was hanged, drawn and quartered, and his wife Margaret Stafford was burnt at the stake. In total, 216 were executed: several lords and knights, six abbots, 38 monks, and sixteen parish priests.

Ten years before the rebellion, Henry was troubled by an ulcer on his left leg. By 1537, he was troubled by ulcers on both legs. The ulcers had become infected and were seeping. The pain started to affect Henry's ability to travel and do the activities he enjoyed. The portrait of Henry, painted by Hans Holbein the Younger in 1537, shows a very different Henry than his previous portraits.

LETTERS FROM COURT

On 30 April 1537, John Husee wrote to Lord Lisle, "As he professes to be your friend I cannot speak to the King; for, as you have scarcely one assured friend to speak in your behalf, you may perchance put him in hazard of losing, or else lose him altogether. When Kyngston spoke to him he made him the same answer as to me. The King goes seldom abroad because his leg is something sore; therefore, you had better speak to Brian on his return, who has for influence no fellow in the Privy Chamber."[142]

On 12 June 1537, Henry wrote to the Duke of Norfolk, "Thus we have declared to you the causes that have specially moved us to put off our intended journey, which you are to set forth as above expressed. But to be frank with you, which you must keep to yourself, a humour has fallen into our legs, and our physicians advise us not to go so far in the heat of the year, even for this reason only."[143]

Treatments from the Tudor Period

The many treatments within the works of his physicians show that Henry continued to be troubled by ulcers. This possible treatment for Henry's ulcers includes the metal mercury, but in a different form than was used in many mercury treatments.[144] I make this distinction because many of the scholars studying the health issues of Henry tried to determine if he was troubled by syphilis, and it was shown that mercury used to treat syphilis was never bought by his household, at least not that could be found.[145]

Dioscorides writes of quicksilver's use, and what is very interesting is that an ingredient used so often to treat syphilis was known as far back as the 1st century AD to be a poison, and he includes what was believed to be a treatment for mercury poisoning:

"It is also found in places where silver is smelted, gathered together in drops on the roofs. Some say that quicksilver is found by itself in the mines. It is kept in glass, lead, tin or silver jars for it eats through all other matter and runs out. It is destructive. Taken as a drink it eats through the internal organs by its weight. This is helped if a lot of milk is taken as a drink, or wine with wormwood, a decoction of smallage, seeds of *Salvia horminum*, *origanum*, or hyssop with wine. (Gold dust, that is, the smallest scraping, is a miraculous help for *hydrargyrum* poisoning)." The following treatment is from Bullein's *Bulwarke of Defence*.

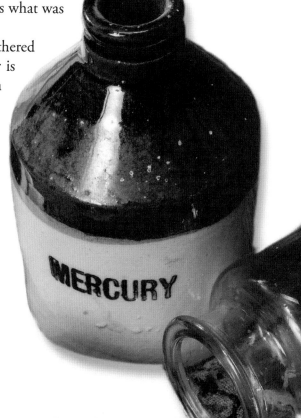

ULCER TREATMENT
- BULLEIN'S BULWARKE OF DEFENCE -
WILLIAM BULLEIN

"

What is the nature of Quickesiluer?

There is mutch variety wheather it should be hoat or colde in the .4 degree, but it should seeme rather to be hoat, by reason it doth dissolue and pearce: it hath vertue to consume, and it is perillous to be vsed in oyntments to kill scabbes with all, for it is percing, and subtill, that at length it will come into the inwarde partes, where as finally it will mortify and kill. It is founde in Minerals of Syluer, and is a destroyer of other mettals. Wyth this Quickesiluer and Sal Armoniake, is made Mercury sublimate, whych must bee kept in a close vessel, adusted in a Ouen, or burnt vntill it come to the couler of whyte Suger, whych Mercury sublimate is vsed of Chirurgians for to cleanse foule vlcers and soares, and is a poyson inwardly to be taken, except with al speede after the same a vomet be taken of Oyle or Azarabaccha[146]

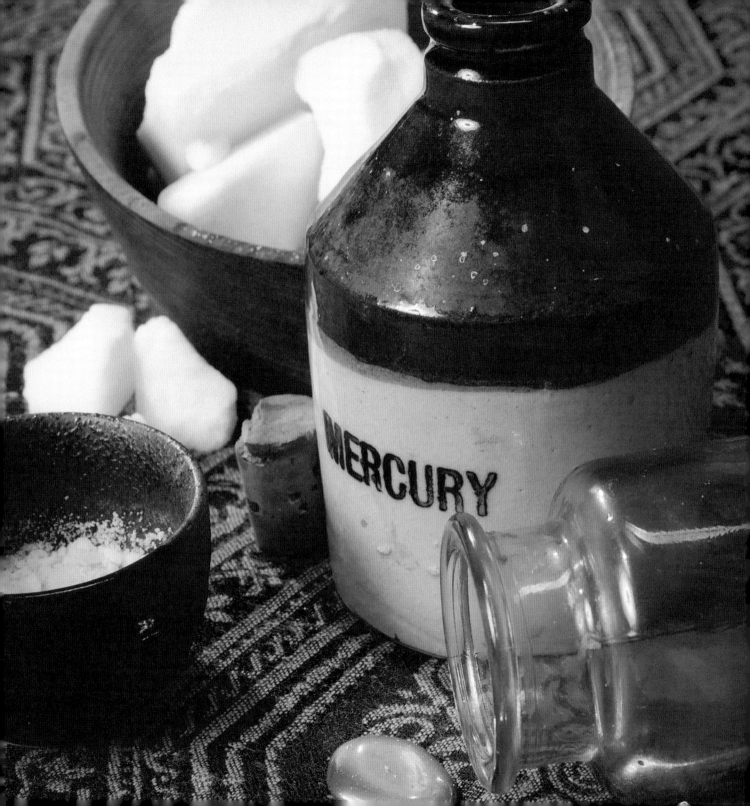

"What is the nature of Quicksilver?

There is much variety whether it should be hot or cold in the 4th degree, but it should seem rather to be hot, by reason it does dissolve and pierce: it hath virtue to consume, and it is perilous to be used in ointments to kill scabs with all, for it is piercing, and subtle, that at length it will come into the inward parts, whereas finally it will mortify and kill. It is found in Minerals of Silver, and is a destroyer of other metals. With this Quicksilver and Sal Ammoniac, is made Mercury sublimate, which must be kept in a closed vessel, adjusted in an Oven, or burnt until it come to the color of white Sugar, which Mercury sublimate is used of Chirurgeons for to cleanse foul ulcers and sores, and is a poison inwardly to be taken, except with all speed after the same a vomit be taken of Oil of Asarabacca"[147]

Mercury sublimate is made with metallic mercury, also called quicksilver, and Sal Ammoniac. Sal Ammoniac is a mineral composed of ammonium chloride and was used into the 1800s to treat wounds. The mixture must be kept in a closed vessel, put in an oven, or burnt until it comes to the colour of white sugar. This physical change to the mercury, by heating and bonding with the Sal Ammoniac, makes it mercury sublimate. Apothecaries and physicians used it to cleanse foul ulcers and sores, but knew it was a poison if taken internally.

It is known that there are some adverse effects from exposure to mercury. "The nervous system is very sensitive to all forms of mercury... Exposure to high levels of metallic, inorganic, or organic mercury can permanently damage the brain, kidneys, and developing foetus. Effects on brain functioning may result in irritability, shyness, tremors, changes in vision or hearing, and memory problems."[148] It is probable that mercury was used to treat ulcers because it was a common treatment for syphilis, and the visible symptoms of syphilis include ulcer-like lesions.

1537/38
FISTULA

In 1537, the "love of Henry's life," Jane Seymour passed away after giving him the son he desired. The year 1538 saw more abbeys dissolved; in fact, over a hundred abbeys, friaries, and priories in that year alone. Eastminster, Wymondham Abbey, Lenton Priory and Austin Friary were all included in the 1538 dissolution. It seemed that just as the abbeys crumbled so did Henry's life.

During the jousting accident in 1536, the horse had fallen on his leg, and it never truly healed. The wound was reopened to drain with a red-hot poker, and developed into a fistula.[149] In the treason trial of the Marquis of Exeter and Lord Montagu, witnesses were called forward to testify that they disrespectfully discussed Henry's health. They said, 'he has a sorre legge that no pore man would be glad off, and that he should not lyve long for all his auctoryte next God' and 'he will die suddenly, his legge will kill him, and then we shall have jolly stirring.'[150]

LETTERS FROM COURT

The French ambassador, the Sieur de Castillon, wrote to the Duke of Montmorency on 14 May 1538, "This King has had stopped one of the fistulas of his legs, and for 10 or 12 days the humours which had no outlet were like to have stifled him, so that he was sometime without speaking, black in the face, and in great danger. God knows if that cheered (a ouvert les esprits) the Lords here, seeing the things that would supervene in such a case. There would be much folly, and my Lord would not be safe if he did not quickly cross the sea. They dare show so little what they think that I only know things by halves. I hear, however, that one party is for the young prince, and the other for Madame Mary. But the King is now so well that no one ever expected it. Norfolk is more welcome than he has been for a long time, and my Lord is suspected for his great Spanish passion. If you think this King should be entertained, we can lead him as you think good, and when, as I write to the King, he has only us as friends, he must come to reason. Would God tho Pope had done him some turn to which he thought the Emperor was consenting; or if we made him amorous there is no better way to catch him. Please think over all I have written, and make me a pasty of it. I will take pains to add whatever sauce you command."[151]

Later that year, when Sir Geoffrey Pole was interrogated by the Crown, it is recorded that "... he seyd that thoughe the Kyng gloryed with the tytylle to be Supreme Hede next God, yet he had a sore lege that no pore man wold be glad off, and that he shold not lyve long for all his auctoryte next God."[152]

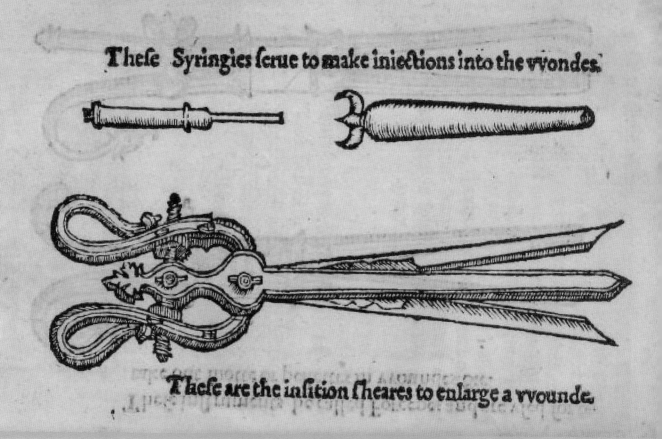

These Syringies serue to make iniections into the vvondes.

These are the insition sheares to enlarge a vvounde.

The image above is taken from Thomas Gale's *Certaine Workes of Chirurgerie*. The woodcut shows two possible tools used on Henry's fistula. The tools at the top are syringes "to make injections into the wounds." These liquid decoctions were used to flush the wounds and it was believed that they helped heal the wound. On the bottom are "insition shears" used to enlarge a wound and open it up. This allowed the fluxes to drain and balance the humours within the wound.

FISTULA TREATMENT
- HENRY'S PRESCRIPTION BOOK -
HENRY VIII AND HIS PHYSICIANS

"

Emplastru flos vnguentorum

Take hartes suett iiij vnces - Rosyn perosin of eche half an pounde, white waxe, frankensense of eche iiij unces. mastique one vnce first mesle the hartes suytt, and the waxe toguether, Then pouldre the gumes, and putt therto, and when they be relented all to guether, strayne them thorough a pece of canvas into a nother vessell, and putt thereto a potell of white wyne, and sett it over the fyre agayn, and boyle them to the consumyng of the wyne. allwayes styrring wt a staff. Then take it frome the fyre, and when it is almost colde, put therto iiij vnces of fyne therebintyne well washed wt white wyne, and ij drames of camphere well powldered. Then make it vpp in rolles, and wrappe them in pchement, This plastre is goode for woundes both newe and olde for brusers, and for achers and it doyth mundifie ulcers and old sores wtout payne, and woll comforte the men ...[illegible due to water spot] on, and is goode both for fistulas and for causes that be ulcerate[153]

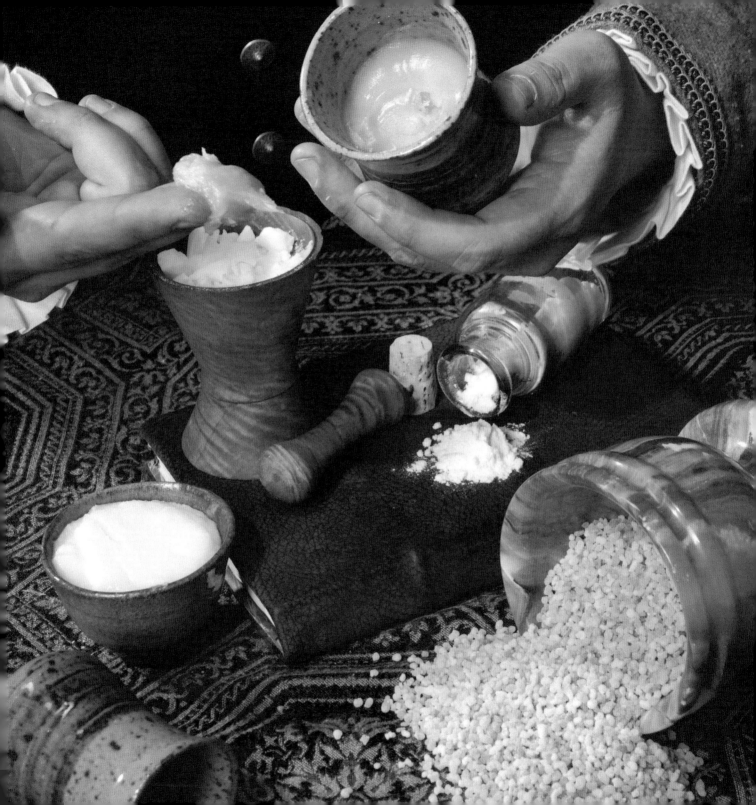

"Emplastru[m] flos vnguentorum

Take hart's suet four ounces – rosin, perosin of each half a pound, white wax, frankincense of each 4 ounces. mastic one ounce. First mesle[154] the hart's suet, and the wax together, then powder the gums, and put thereto, and when they be relented all together, strain them thorough a piece of canvas into another vessel, and put thereto a potelle of white wine, and set it over the fire again, and boil them to the consuming of the wine. always stirring with a staff. Then take it from the fire, and when it is almost cold, put thereto four ounces of fine turpentine well washed with white wine, and two drams of camphor well powdered. Then make it up in rolls, and wrap them in parchment, this plaster is good for wounds both new and old for bruises, and for aches and it does mundifie[155] ulcers and old sores without pain, and will comfort the men[…] on, and is good both for fistulas and for causes that be ulcerate"

To treat a fistula, I chose "Emplastrum flos vnguentorum" from the *Prescription book of Henry VIII*. To make the plaster, take four ounces of hart's suet, also known as deer tallow, half a pound each of rosin and perosin, or resin from a pear tree, four ounces each of white wax and frankincense, and one ounce of mastic, resin from the mastic tree. Heat and mix the tallow and wax together, then add the gums, after they have been powdered. When they are all mixed together, strain them through a piece of canvas into another vessel. Put in a half gallon of white wine, and set it on the fire again, and boil and continue to stir until the wine has evaporated. Then take it from the heat, and when it is almost cold, mix in four ounces of fine turpentine and two drams of camphor, that has been powdered. Then make it up in rolls, and wrap them in parchment and save for use. The physicians of Henry wrote that this treatment is "good both for fistulas and for causes that be ulcerate."

John Gerard wrote in his 1597 herbal that rosin and turpentine are hot and dry, are "an astringent" and are "cleansing"[156] He also said that mastic is more of an astringent but less cleaning than rosin. Dioscorides writes of the uses of frankincense, "It is able to warm and is an astringent to clean away things which darken the pupils, fill up the hollowness of ulcers and draw them to a scar, and to glue together bloody wounds; and it is able to suppress all excessive discharges of blood including that of the neural membrane. Pounded into small pieces and applied with linen dipped in milk it lessens malignant ulcers around the perineum and other parts."[157] The fifth ingredient that is warming is camphor and Dioscorides says, "It warms, and is effective rubbed on for those things that darken the pupils, and daubed on is good for leprosy and painful nerves."[158] All of the herbal ingredients in this treatment were selected for their warming effect, and indicate that the physicians thought that the humours were out of balance and that this caused the fistula.

Henry's fistula was the last of the major illnesses that affected him up until his major decline and death ten years later. The last few months of his life are not included in this book. The king had so many complaints[159] and there were many physicians all trying to keep the king alive, that it would take a book of its own. There is one more ailment to examine and, while compared to fistulas or ulcers it may not seem like a huge deal, any who have been troubled by constipation know that it can be quite uncomfortable and even painful.

1539
CONSTIPATION

12 January 1539 found Henry's ability to form alliances constricted. Charles V, the Holy Roman Emperor, and Francis I of France signed the Treaty of Toledo. Through this treaty, the kings agreed to make no more alliances with the Kingdom of England. Charles was Holy Roman Emperor, King of Spain, King of the Romans, King of Italy, Lord of the Netherlands, and Duke of Burgundy, with France included by the Treaty of Toledo. Henry had few kingdoms to rely on. However, it was not just Henry's ability to form international relations that was constipated.

Modern people do not like talking about using the bathroom, and especially avoid talking about issues with constipation, haemorrhoids or diarrhoea. The king, however, had no privacy, and his movements were never inconspicuous. In fact, he had a "Groom of the Stool" who oversaw his most private business. In 1539, his constipation appeared to be more than just a minor issue, and the issues were recorded by the most intimate of his courtiers.

During Henry's 36-year reign, he had four Grooms of the Stool. From 1509 to 1526 the role was taken by Sir William Compton. Sir William was knighted during this time and also acted as an Under-Treasurer of the Exchequer, Chancellor of Ireland and sheriff of a few regions. After Sir William, came Sir Henry Norris, who was Groom of the Stool for ten years. His term ended with his execution as one of the four men found guilty with Queen Anne Boleyn. Sir Thomas Heneage then held the office for a decade, followed by Sir Anthony Denny for just two years, as the king passed away in 1547.

LETTERS FROM COURT

"I received your letter this morning, although your servant came over night; 'for by th'advice of the physicians the King's Majesty went betimes to bed, whose Highness slept until two of the clock in the morning, and then his Grace rose to go to the stool which, by working of the pills and glister[160] that his Highness had taken before, had a very fair siege, as the said physicians have made report; not doubting but the worst is past by their perseverance, to no danger of any further grief to remain in him, and the hinder part of the night until 10 of the clock this morning his Grace had very good rest, and his Grace findeth himself well, saving his Highness saith he hath a little soreness in his body. And I would have had his said Majesty to have read your letter, but would that I should make to him relation thereof, whereat his Grace smiled, saying that your Lordship had much more fear than required.' I will send your bills as soon as his Grace has signed them. The long tarrying of your servant here was by my command. Hampthill, Friday, between 10 and 11 a.m."[161]

With the diet that Henry ate, it is no wonder that he had some digestive issues. Henry, of course, was not the only one eating at the Tudor court. In one year, meat consumption totalled 1,240 oxen, 8,200 sheep, 2,330 deer, 760 calves, 1,870 pigs and 53 wild boars and they drank 600,000 gallons of beer.[162] *A Declaracion of the Particular Ordinances of Fares for the Dietts to be served to the King's Highnesse, the Queen's Grace, and the sides, with the Household*[163] shows that an awful lot of meat and not enough fibre were consumed at Henry VIII's court. It is no wonder he was troubled by constipation.

GLYSTER
- BULLEIN'S BULWARKE OF DEFENCE -
WILLIAM BULLEIN

"

What vertue is in the herbe Rumex, called the great Docke, I meane not the Sorel, called Acedula, wherof you answered mee before in this booke.

I Knowe your meaning very well, of that wilde herbe, whych groweth commonly by pathes, hedges, and waters sides. And of this kynd, ther is one called Monkes Rubarbe, which groweth in gardens, the other is wilde and with lesser leaues. Marcellus, the blynd ignoraunt people, haue of long tyme not a little erred, in one kynd of Lappa or Rumex. I meane neither Sorell, nor the common wyld Docke, or the bastard Rubarbe: but that which is commonly called Mercurie, with golden sandes, vppon the back sydes of the leaues, great rootes, clusters of seedes, leaues like a brode speare head, not purfled about with iagges, or smal teeth like a saw, which in deede the very Mercurie hath, with one onely roote. Whereupon many small fine rootes do grow, like a bush: and thys Mercurie is mutch like vnto wylde Hempe. But this bastard Mercurie, whereof I haue now spoken called Rumex, is none other but a kynd of Dockes, which being sodden, or vsed in Clyster, wil moue the belly to bee laxatiue. And is good to be sodden in brothes for them which haue the yellow Iaundice.[164]

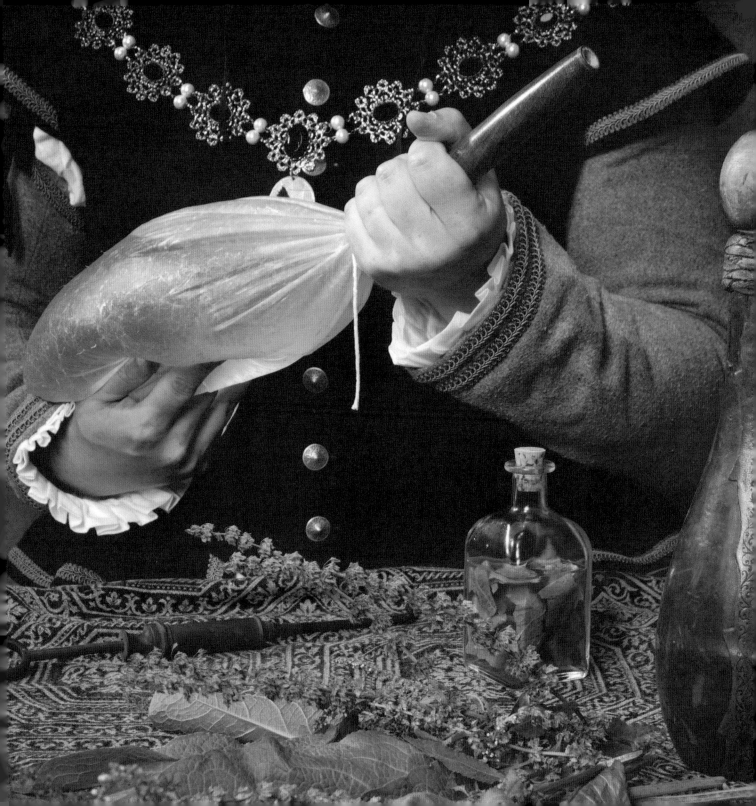

"What virtue is in the herb Rumex, called the great Dock, I mean not the Sorrel, called Acedula, whereof you answered me before in this book.

I know your meaning very well, of that wild herb, which grows commonly by paths, hedges, and waters sides. And of this kind, there is one called Monks Rhubarb, which grows in gardens, the other is wild and with lesser leaves. Marcellus, the blind ignorant people, have of long time not a little erred, in one kind of Lappa or Rumex. I mean neither Sorrel, nor the common wild Dock, or the bastard Rhubarb: but that which is commonly called Mercury, with golden sands, upon the back sides of the leaves, great roots, clusters of seeds, leaves like a broad spear head, not purfled about with jaggs, or small teeth like a saw, which in deed the very Mercury hath, with one only root. Whereupon many small fine roots do grow, like a bush: and this Mercury is much like unto wild Hemp. But this bastard mercury, whereof I have now spoken called Rumex, is none other but a kind of Dock, which being sodden, or used in Clyster,[165] will move the belly to be laxative. And is good to be sodden in broths for them which have the yellow Jaundice"

Bullein talks of using dock, a broad-leaved wayside plant with large tap-roots, or rumex, for a glyster being sodden. He says it will move the belly to be laxative. The fluid for the glister should be made like a decoction, or boiled mash, and the plant product strained from the remaining water. Then the fluid is placed in the pig bladder, another bag, or a syringe. The bag is attached to a tube and the tube inserted into the rectum. The bag is then squeezed, forcing the fluid into the rectum.

Dioscorides wrote about the types of dock and that "all of these (boiled) soothe the intestines."[169] However, the process of an enema without a herb or chemical other than a natural saline, will have a desired effect just by filling the rectum with fluid, expanding out the walls of the rectum, and making it easier for the stool to move

When researching this treatment, I assumed that the dock had little to do with the treatment, however, on further investigation, I found that it contains anthraquinone.[170] "Besides their utilization as colourants, anthraquinone derivatives have been used for centuries for medical applications, for example, as laxatives and antimicrobial and anti-inflammatory agents. Current therapeutic indications include constipation, arthritis, multiple sclerosis, and cancer."[171] It appears that this treatment, along with the laxative pills on the next page, could very well have been the reason for Henry's "very fair siege."

Laxative Pills
- Bullein's Bulwarke of Defence -
William Bullein

"

How make you Pilles of Fumiterre.

TAke of the fyue kyndes of Mirobalans, ana. ʒ.v. of Aloes. ʒ.vi. of
Scammony. ʒ.v. mingle them with the iuice of Fumiterre, and let them
stand til they bee dry, then sprinckle on agayne the iuice of Fumiterre,
and suffer them agayne, to drye and so do the thyrd tyme, then let
them stand vntill they bee thicke, and then make your pilles. [166]

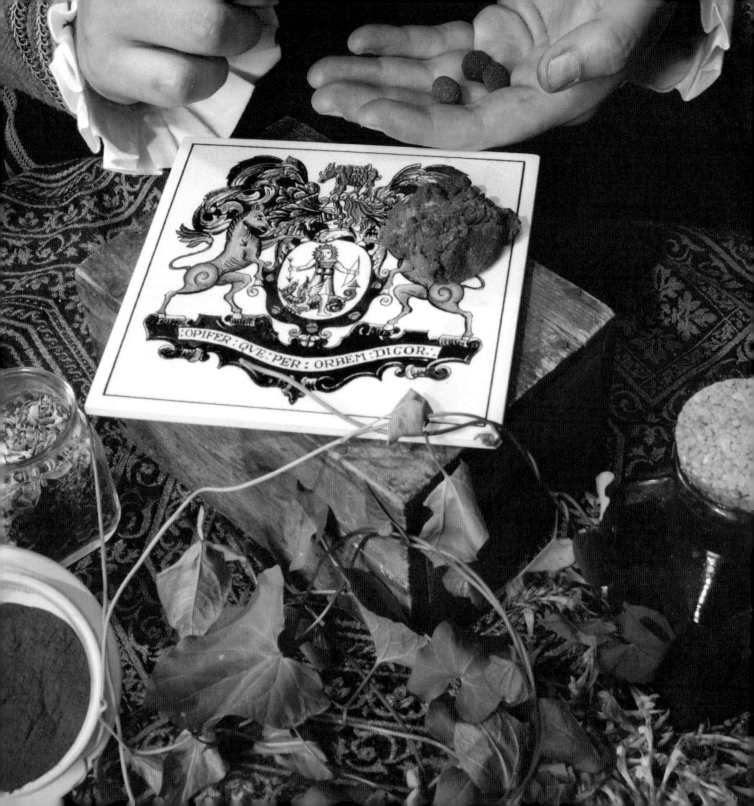

"How to make your Pills of Fumiterre.

Take five kinds of Myrobalans and use 5 drams, 6 drams of Aloe, 5 drams of Scammony, and mix them with the juice of Fumiterre. Let them stand till they are dry, then sprinkle on again the juice of Fumiterre, and suffer them again to dry, and do it again a third time. Then let them stand until they are thick, and then make your pills."

From the passage by Henry's Chamberlain of the Stool we know that Henry took a pill, as well as using a glyster for his constipation. William Bullein refers to a purgation called "pilles de fumo terrae," and, later in his book, he says how to make them. Take the five kinds of Myrobalans, Aloe and Scammony, a plant in the morning glory family, and mix them with the juice of Fume Terre, an annual plant, with grey-green leaves, and tube-like flowers and let them stand till they are dry. Then sprinkle more juice of Fume Terre, and let dry and do so two times, then let them stand until they are thick, and then make your pills.

Dioscorides wrote about myrobalan, "It has strength to clean spots, freckles, down on the face, and darkening cataracts and it purges the intestines."[167] In *De Materia Medica* it is also written, "To loosen the bowels twenty grains are enough, taken with sesame or some other seed. For more effective purging thirty grains of the juice is given with twenty grains of black hellebore and one teaspoonful of aloe. Purging salts are prepared with twenty teaspoonfuls of the juice of scammony mixed with six cups of salt."[168] This means that myrobalan, scammony, and aloe have both been used since the 1st century AD to purge the bowels.

CONCLUSION

The examination of seventeen treatments used by Tudor physicians is an eye-opening experience. It is amazing that those born in 16th century England had the average life expectancy of around 35, with a much higher average if they survived to adulthood. With lead-based topical treatments, mercuric ulcer treatments, and blood-letting, it is safe to say that a treatment might often have done more harm than the original sickness. While we do not know with all certainty that Henry was treated with these treatments, it is likely that even if they were not exactly as written by his physicians, they will have been similar. The medical theories of the Tudor period, originally from over a millennium before, as well as many of the alleged uses of herbs, derived from herbals 1500 years old, would dictate the treatments to be similar to those studied. Either way, we can use these treatments as a starting point to delve deeper into Tudor medicine, see pre-modern medical practices in use, make the scrutiny of medical texts feel a little more human, and see some additional possible reasons for the actions of one of England's most infamous rulers.

Some areas for further research include any of the primary sources for treatments: the physicians themselves, herbals like William Turners *A New Herball*, or Gerard's *A History of Plants*, and the treatments made by Henry's Gentlemen Apothecary, listed in "Letters and Papers". Each of the texts written by Henry's physicians is filled with numerous treatments, and includes the first English reference to gunshot wounds, or a look at illnesses, like sweating sickness, whose causes are still unknown today. I recommend that those that want to delve deeper, start with reading though Thomas Gale or William Bullein's texts. By doing this, you can start to see what the physicians saw. The herbals written in the 1500s in England, as well as numerous earlier herbals that were published with the invention of the printing press the century before, are treasure troves of information, and windows into the ideas of the members of the medical community. The lists of items made by Thomas

Alsop, and charged to Henry, include items made for the household as well as for Henry himself. The bill is an interesting source of what type of daily items were made for a royal household, like "perfumes for the Closet," "sugar candy and mell. ross. for the hawks," and "pills of mastick and aqua caprifolii."

While Henry VIII's jousting accident has often been blamed for his change from a Renaissance Prince, praised by many across Europe, to an irrational tyrant by the end of his reign, it was not the only thing that could have affected his personality. I think that one part of the issue is the stress on the royals, to secure the line of succession, constant reminders from advisors and pressure to have a son. Not that this is in anyway an excuse for the horrible treatment of the women in his life. I also believe that chronic pain from the fistula was an immense factor in Henry's moods. Working in the medical field myself, it is easy to see a correlation between those with chronic pain and mood changes. Finally, and I feel the least examined possibility, is the actual treatments that Tudor physicians used to treat disease. Many of the treatments used heavy metals, and we now know the effects those metals have on our bodies and minds.

To understand the reasoning behind physicians from the 16th century picking a treatment, we took a brief look at the theories of the day regarding diagnosing and prescribing. Humoral theory, doctrine of signatures, uroscopy and astrological theory were all used in the 16th century to assist a physician. Though modern medicine has found all these invalid, they were commonly used and even required by law into the 1800s. Taking a deeper look at these theories, as well as connecting them, through the medical texts of Henry's physicians, to a real person with tangible ailments, we see a science more humanized.

The medical staff of Henry VIII of England left gaps in his medical history, because the records have been lost or destroyed, or Henry VIII's physicians did not keep records of what they did to treat Henry, possibly for their own protection. We filled these gaps by first finding references to his illnesses in letters from his court, then analysing works written by Henry's physicians to determine what Tudor physicians would have done to treat the various illnesses. Using the medical texts of Henry's medical staff, I recreated some of the identified treatments, and I examined the ingredients to look at the history of their uses through early medical texts, and at the harmful effects that could have happened because of our knowledge now of modern medicine and science. This was a case study, the study of a person over a period of time, not only to present possible treatments for an infamous ruler, but to open a window into the world of Tudor medicine.

Seamus O'Caellaigh

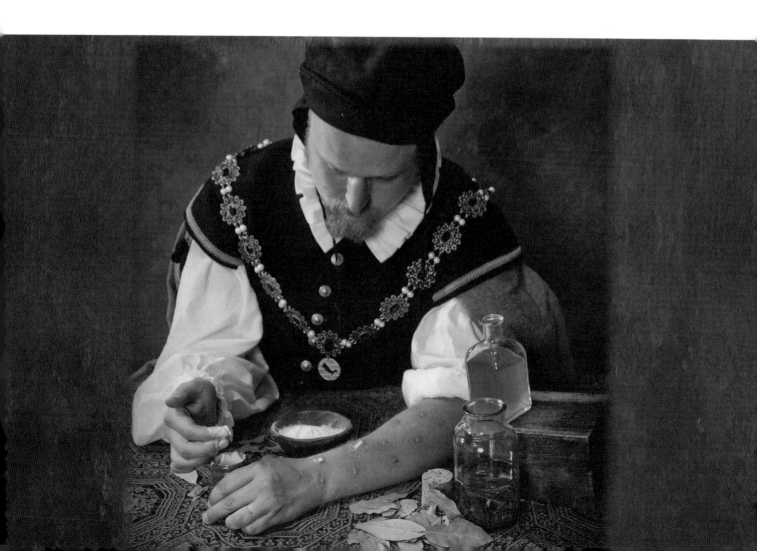

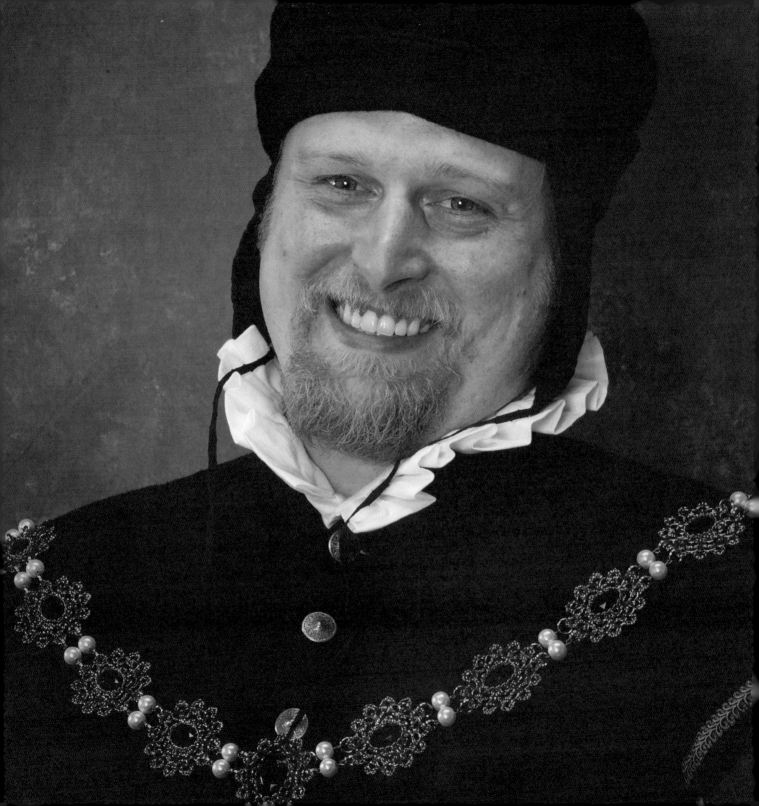

Seamus O'Caellaigh has always been interested in the Tudor dynasty and the many uses of plants. He grew up learning about plants from his grandmother Anne Kelley and mother Diane Prickett. Their love of plants has manifested in Seamus through his love of being out in the wild looking for medicinal plants, through his spending lots of time in the family garden and through spending time in the woods in the Pacific Northwest. He is most often seen with his head down, looking at the plants along the path and not at what lies ahead.

Having joined a pre-1600s recreation group, Seamus found a way to incorporate his love of the Tudors with a study of medicinal plants from that time period, along with the many herbal books written from the 1st century to the turn of the 17th century. Nothing makes Seamus happier than finding an obscure reference, or his son Jerrick bringing him a plant for "Dad's Plant Projects."

SPECIAL THANKS

Thank you, Stacey Kelley, David Little, and Jerrick Kelley for putting up with my obsessions daily and my 16th century treatments being all over the house. Without your support, I would have not been able to do this. Speaking of support, my chosen family in the SCA, Whitney Dickinson, Brian Huffman, Trish Graham, Jacob Caspe and Britta Hall, you never wavered in your support. Ashley White and Simone Hanebaum, thank you for being a sounding block, and leading me in my journey of transcribing Tudor handwriting. Finally, the group of people that read and gave feedback, Joe Cook-Giles, Kevin Hodges, Deb Parker, Mary Anne Bartlett, Cynthia Ley, and Laurel Grasmick-Black, thank you does not seem enough. I learned something from each of you and I am more thankful than I can say.

A huge thank you to Vocaleyes Photography for the wonderful pictures! Robert and Janet, you are both amazing artists and made apothecary come alive. I encourage everyone to look at their work on vocaleyes.net. It is truly photography that sings!

BIBLIOGRAPHY

"A History of the Royal Game of Tennis"
Real Tennis History - Tennis & Rackets Association. Accessed April 29, 2017.
https://www.tennisandrackets.com/real-tennis-history.aspx.

Besharat, Sima, Mahsa Besharat, and Ali Jabbari. "Wild lettuce (Lactuca virosa) toxicity."
BMJ Case Reports. 2009. Accessed August 21, 2017. https://www.ncbi.nlm.nih.
gov/pmc/articles/PMC3031874/#b1.

Breverton, Terry. *The Physicians of Myddfai: Cures and Remedies of the Mediaeval World.*
Carmarthen: Cambria Books, 2012.

Bullein, William. *Bullein's bulwarke of defence against all sicknesse, soarenesse, and woundes
that doe dayly assaulte mankinde: which bulwarke is kept with Hilarius the gardener,
& health the physicion, with the chirugian, to helpe the wounded souldiours: Gathered
and practised from the most worthy learned, both olde and new; to the great comfort of
mankinde.* Imprinted at London: By Thomas Marshe, 1579.

Buttes, William , John Chambre, Walter Cromer, and Agostino Degli Agostini.
*Henry VIII of England: Medical receipts devised by the King and the Royal Physicians:
16th century.* Sloane Manuscript 1047.

Cawdrey, Robert. "A Table Alphabeticall of Hard Usual English Words"
(R. Cawdrey, 1604). 1997. Accessed April 27, 2017.
http://library.utoronto.ca/utel/ret/cawdrey/cawdrey0.html.

Chalmers, CR, and EJ Chaloner, "500 Years Later: Henry VIII, Leg Ulcers and the
Course of History", *Journal of the Royal Society of Medicine.* (2009)

Creighton, Charles. *A History of Epidemics in Britain.*
Cambridge: Cambridge University Press, 2013.

Culpeper, Nicholas. *Culpeper's Complete Herbal, and English Physician.* Leicester, UK: Magna Books, 1992.

Dioscorides, Pedanius, T. A. Osbaldeston, and R. P. A. Wood. *Dioscorides de materia medica: being an herbal with many other medicinal materials.* Johannesburg: IBIDIS, 2000.

Elder, Pliny The. *Delphi Ancient Classics: Complete works of Pliny the Elder.* Hastings, East Sussex, UK: Delphi Publishing Limited, 2011.

Emmison, F. G. *Elizabethan Life: Morals & the Church Courts, Mainly from Essex Archidiaconal Records,* Essex County Council, 1973.

"Environmental Health and Medicine Education." Centers for Disease Control and Prevention. August 20, 2007. Accessed April 28, 2017. https://www.atsdr.cdc.gov/csem/csem.asp?csem=7&po=10.

Feis, Julia Rae. "Henry VIII: Patient and Patron of Medicine." Master's thesis, University of Colorado, Boulder , 2013. Spring 2013. Accessed April 23, 2017. http://scholar.colorado.edu/honr_theses/346/.

Francis, John, comp. *Notes & Queries; a Medium of Intercommunication for Literary Men, General Readers, Etc.* Vol. 11. 4th Series. London: Wellington Street, 1873.

Frith, John, "Syphilis – Its Early History and Treatment until Penicillin and the Debate on Its Origins", *JMVH* (2016).

Furdell, Elizabeth Lane. *The Royal Doctors, 1485-1714: Medical Personnel at the Tudor and Stuart Courts.* Rochester, NY: University of Rochester Press, 2001.

Gale, Thomas. *Certaine workes of chirurgerie: Gale, Thomas, 1507-1587.* Internet Archive. February 25, 2011. Accessed April 25, 2017. https://archive.org/details/certainevvorkeso00gale. Original held at Boston Medical Library in the Francis A. Countway Library of Medicine.

Garnett, Richard, and Gosse, Edmund.
  English literature: an illustrated record: in four volumes, Volume 1,
  London: William Heinemann, 1903.

Gerard, John, and Thomas Johnson. *The Herbal or General History of Plants: The
  Complete 1633 Edition as Revised and Enlarged by Thomas Johnson.*
  New York: Dover, 1975.

Giustinian, Sebastian. *Four years at the court of Henry VIII: Selection of despatches written
  by the Venetian Ambassador Sebastian Giustinian, and Addressed to the Signory
  of Venice,* London: Smith, Elder, & Co., 1854.

Hall, Edward. *Hall's chronicle : containing the history of England, during the reign of Henry
  the Fourth, and the succeeding monarchs, to the end of the reign of Henry the Eighth,
  in which are particularly described the manners and customs of those periods. Carefully
  collated with the editions of 1548 and 1550,*
  Internet Archive. January 17, 2007. Accessed August 28, 2017.
  https://archive.org/details/hallschronicleco00halluoft.

"Hampton Court Palace." - *Palaces, Historic Royal Official Website*
  https://www.hrp.org.uk/hampton-court-palace/explore/henry-viiis-kitchens/

Johnston, Carol S., and Cindy A. Gaas. "Vinegar: Medicinal Uses and Antiglycemic
  Effect." *Medscape General Medicine.* May 30, 2006. Accessed January 18, 2017.
  https://www.ncbi.nlm.nih.gov/pmc/articles/PMC1785201/ .

Kramer, Kyra. "Henry VIII: Fit, Fat, Fiction." Lecture. December 17, 2015. Accessed
  October 28, 2017.

Letters and Papers, Foreign and Domestic, Henry VIII. Edited by J S Brewer. London: His
  Majesty's Stationery Office 1920. *British History Online.* Accessed March 2016,
  http://www.british-history.ac.uk/letters-papers-hen8/.

MacNalty, Sir Arthur Salusbury. *Henry VIII: A Difficult Patient,*
  Christopher Johnson, 1952.

Malik, Enas M., and Muller, Christa E., "Anthraquinones As Pharmacological Tools and Drugs", *Medicinal Research Reviews* 36.4 (2016): 705-48. Web. 18 Jan. 2017.

Morris, Terence Alan. *Europe and England in the sixteenth century.* London: Routledge, 1998.

ed. Nichols, John. *A collection of ordinances and regulations for the government of the royal household, made in divers reigns. From King Edward III. to King William and Queen Mary. Also receipts in ancient cookery,* London, Printed for the Society of Antiquaries, 1790.

Noack, Dunja, dir. "Inside the Body of Henry VIII", National Geographic. April 20, 2008.

Scarisbrick, J. J. *Henry VIII.* New Haven: Yale University Press, 2012.

Schilling, Judith A., and Sean Webb. *Nursing Herbal Medicine Handbook.* Philadelphia: Lippincott, Williams & Wilkins, 2006.

Skelton, John. "Elegy on the Death of Henry VII." Accessed April 02, 2017. http://www.otago.ac.nz/english-linguistics/tudor/death_henryvii13075.html.

"Smallpox." Centers for Disease Control and Prevention. September 26, 2016. Accessed January 12, 2017. https://www.cdc.gov/smallpox/

Van Soest, Rob . "Clathria coralloides." Marine Species Identification Portal : Clathria coralloides. Accessed April 28, 2017. http://species-identification.org/species.php?species_group=sponges&id=161&menuentry=soorten.

Weir, Alison. *The Six Wives of Henry VIII.* London: The Bodley Head, 1991.

Wight, Colin. "'Pastime with good company': composition by Henry VIII." The British Library. April 24, 2012. Accessed August 10, 2017. http://www.bl.uk/onlinegallery/onlineex/henryviii/musspowor/pastime/

NOTES

1. Based on the theory that the human body is made up of four fluids.
2. Herbals are books about plants especially regarding their medicinal properties.
3. Dioscorides finished *De Materia Medica* in AD 60. It was first printed in 1478 (in Anderson, Frank J. *An Illustrated History of the Herbals*), 15.
4. Elizabeth Lane Furdell, *The Royal Doctors, 1485-1714: Medical Personnel at the Tudor and Stuart Courts*, 85.
5. A plant based drug having only one ingredient.
6. Made up of two or more parts.
7. Theriac, originally called *Mithridatium*, created in the 1st century BC and used to prevent poisoning, grew through the Middle Ages and Renaissance to contain sometimes as many as 70 ingredients, and was used to treat plague, poisoning and any number of illnesses. It was considered a cure-all as was even sold as such up to the 1980s.
8. Part of the great collection of manuscripts and artefacts gathered by the physician Sir Hans Sloane (1660-1753) and purchased at his death from his executors by the Act of Parliament which also established the British Museum.
9. Furdell, 25.
10. Buttes, Chambre, Cromer, and Agostini. *Henry VIII of England: Medical receipts devised by the King and the Royal Physicians: 16th century.* Sloane Manuscript 1047.
11. Furdell, 26.
12. *Letters and Papers, Foreign and Domestic, Henry VIII, Volume 1, 1509-1514*, 2686.
13. Charles Creighton, *A History of Epidemics in Britain*, 450.

14. Sebastian Giustinian, *Four years at the court of Henry VIII: Selection of despatches written by the Venetian Ambassador Sebastian Giustinian, and Addressed to the Signory of Venice*, 47.

15. *Letters and Papers, Volume 1*, 2703.

16. Ibid., 2697.

17. John Francis, comp. *Notes & Queries; a Medium of Intercommunication for Literary Men, General Readers, Etc.* Vol. 11. 4th Series, 54.

18. "Smallpox." Centers for Disease Control and Prevention.

19. Ibid.

20. Ibid.

21. Bullein, "The Booke of Simples", Folio 28.

22. A tisane of barley water.

23. One of the four bodily humours, identified with bile and believed to be associated with a peevish or irascible temperament.

24. Dioscorides, Pedanius, T. A. Osbaldeston, and R. P. A. Wood. *Dioscorides de materia medica: being an herbal with many other medicinal materials*, Book 2, 230

25. Bullein, "The Booke of Simples", Folio 28.

26. A plant species from the genus *Hyssopus* and the family *Lamiaceae*.

27. A plant species from the genus *Ruta* and the family *Rutaceae*,

28. A strong, sweet white wine imported from Greece and the eastern Mediterranean islands.

29. Resin, especially the solid amber residue obtained after the distillation of crude turpentine *oleoresin*, or of naphtha extract from pine stumps.

30. A plant species from the genus *Chelidonium* and of the family *Papaveraceae*.

31. The region of the thorax immediately in front of or over the heart.

32. A plant species from the genus *Melilotus* and of the family *Fabaceae*.

33. While Dioscorides wrote his herbal in the 1st century it was referenced in medical texts until the 1800s.

34. Dioscorides, Book 2, 292.

35. The plant species *Lactuca virosa* from the family *Asteraceae*.
36. Dioscorides, Book 4. 607
37. The outer layer of a plant, like a skin.
38. Sima Besharat, Mahsa Besharat, and Ali Jabbari. "Wild lettuce (Lactuca virosa) toxicity".
39. Bullein, "The Booke of Simples", Folio 69.
40. A province in northern central Italy.
41. Bullein, "The Booke of Simples", Folio 69.
42. Culpeper, *Culpeper's Complete Herbal, and English Physician*, 214.
43. Air swallowed while eating, or gas generated in the stomach and intestines by digestion.
44. Culpeper, 13.
45. A bacterial skin infection.
46. A skin disease with red pustules.
47. A membrane on an eye.
48. Dioscorides, Book 5, 754.
49. Carol S. Johnston and Cindy A. Gaas. "Vinegar: Medicinal Uses and Antiglycemic Effect."
50. Dioscorides, Book 5, 807.
51. Pliny the Elder, *Delphi ancient classics: Complete works of Pliny the Elder*, Book XXVIII, Chapter 7.
52. *Letters and Papers, Foreign and Domestic, Henry VIII, Volume 3, 1519-1523*, 1233.
53. Ibid., 1245
54. A poem, typically mourning the dead.
55. John Skelton, "Elegy on the Death of Henry VII.", spelling modernised by the author.
56. Consumption is a wasting disease, likely tuberculosis.
57. An unknown disease characterized as having fevers with intense sweating, epidemic in England in the 15ᵗʰ–16ᵗʰ centuries.

58. *Letters and Papers, Foreign and Domestic, Henry VIII, Volume 3, 1519-1523*, 1293.

59. Ibid, 1306.

60. Ibid, 1308

61. "Malaria" Centers for Disease Control and Prevention.

62. Murky, opaque, or thick with precipitates.

63. Terry Breverton, *The Physicians of Myddfai: Cures and Remedies of the Mediaeval World*, 101.

64. Bullein, "The Booke of Simples", Folio 35.

65. Culpeper stated that there are two categories of oil: simple and compound. Compound oils are made by a carrier oil absorbing the virtues of a flower, herb or leaves.

66. John Gerard and Thomas Johnson, *The Herbal or, General History of Plants: The complete 1633 edition as revised and enlarged by Thomas Johnson*, 588.

67. A Medieval joust or spear play.

68. Colin Wight, *Pastime with good company': composition by Henry VIII*; Richard Garnett and Edmund Gosse, *English Literature: an illustrated record: in four volumes*, Volume 1, 357

69. A kingdom in the Northeastern part of the Spanish Peninsula.

70. *Letters and Papers, Foreign and Domestic, Henry VIII, Volume 4, 1524*, 771.

71. Edward Hall, *Hall's chronicle : containing the history of England, during the reign of Henry the Fourth, and the succeeding monarchs, to the end of the reign of Henry the Eighth, in which are particularly described the manners and customs of those periods.*

72. Thomas Gale, *Certaine workes of chirurgerie*, "The Second Booke of the Enchiridion", 18-19.

73. To make flesh.

74. To heal by scar formation.

75. A soft greasy or viscous substance used as ointment.

76. Related to the Greek word *Penos* meaning web.

77. To mix, mingle, combine, blend.

78. Having the power to cleanse (especially an ulcer or wound).
79. Culpeper, 214.
80. Ibid.
81. Claudius Galenus (born AD 130).
82. Assuage - Making an unpleasant feeling less intense.
83. Gerard, 1264.
84. "A History of the Royal Game of Tennis,"
85. *Letters and Papers, Foreign and Domestic, Henry VIII, Volume 3, 1519-1523*, 402
86. To injure (a part of the body) as a result of a sudden twisting movement, *Oxford Dictionaries*.
87. Feis, "Henry VIII: Patient and Patron of Medicine,"
88. Scarisbrick, *Henry VIII*, 44.
89. Morris, *Europe and England in the sixteenth century*, 151.
90. Gale, "The Fourthe Booke of the Enchiridion", 51
91. Dislocated.
92. A long surgical bandage rolled up for ease of application.
93. (980–1037), Persian-born Islamic philosopher and physician; Arabic name ibn-Sina. His philosophical system, drawing on Aristotle but in many ways closer to Neoplatonism, was the major influence on the development of scholasticism. His "Canon of Medicine" was a standard medieval medical text.
94. Covered with wax or resin.
95. Gale, "The Fourthe Booke of the Enchiridion", 51.
96. Both physical and mental pain or distress.
97. Of varying types; several.
98. A book containing essential information on a subject.
99. Cutting of a vein.
100. The operation of cutting into or opening an artery (in early use especially for blood-letting).
101. Make shallow incisions in (the skin), especially as a medical procedure.

102. Noack, "Inside the Body of Henry VIII".
103. Inflammation of bone or bone marrow, usually due to infection.
104. Kramer, "Henry VIII: Fit, Fat, Fiction".
105. Emmison.
106. Gale.
107. Become larger or stronger.
108. Reduce to a smaller size.
109. A polysaccharide substance extracted as a viscous or gelatinous solution from plant roots, seeds, etc., and used in medicines and adhesives.
110. Overlapping.
111. *Althaea officinalis* from the mallow family.
112. Resin from the plant *Dorema ammoniacum* of the family *Apiaceae*.
113. Resin from the plant *Daemomorops draco*.
114. "Environmental Health and Medicine Education".
115. Dioscorides, Book 5, 783.
116. Buttes, Chambre, Cromer, and Agostini.
117. Flowers of the genus *Diospyros*.
118. Any of several plants of the family *Gentianaceae*.
119. Schilling and Webb, 68.
120. Ibid., 104.
121. Bullein, Book of Simples, Fol. 62.
122. Mesue the Elder, Persian Physician (777AD – 857AD).
123. A plant of the *convolvulus* family, the dried roots of which yield a strong purgative.
124. Dioscorides, Book 4, 715.
125. Chalmers and Chaloner.
126. *Letters and Papers, Foreign and Domestic, Henry VIII, Volume 10, 1536*, 200.
127. Ibid., 294.
128. Gale, "The Firste Booke of the Enchiridion", 9-10.
129. A flowering plant from the genus *Gentiana*.

130. Having the power to cleanse.
131. Rolled Bandages.
132. Formless.
133. Resin from the Mastic tree, *Pistacia lentiscus*.
134. Root from iris species *Iris germanica* or *Iris pallida*.
135. The two most common plantains are *Plantago major* and *Plantago minor*.
136. Gale, "The Firste Booke of the Enchiridion", 11.
137. Made from verdigris, vinegar, and honey
138. A colourless astringent compound which is a hydrated double sulphate of aluminium and potassium, used in solution in dyeing and tanning.
139. Culpeper.
140. An uprising in October 1536 due to Henry's breaking with the Roman Catholic Church and Dissolution of the Monasteries.
141. *Letters and Papers, Foreign and Domestic, Henry VIII, Volume 12 Part 1,* 1227.
142. Ibid., 1068.
143. *Letters and Papers, Foreign and Domestic, Henry VIII, Volume 12 Part 2,* 77.
144. Frith.
145. Chalmers and Chaloner.
146. Bullein, "The Booke of Simples", Fol. 69.
147. A wild ginger, botanically called *Asarum europaeum*.
148. "Mercury Exposure", *CDC: Centers for Disease Control and Prevention*.
149. A fistula is a dangerous ulcer or running sore.
150. Chalmers and Chaloner.
151. *Letters and Papers, Foreign and Domestic, Henry VIII, Volume 13 Part 1,* 995.
152. *Letters and Papers, Foreign and Domestic, Henry VIII, Volume 13 Part 2,* 800.
153. Buttes, Chambre, Cromer, and Agostini.
154. To mingle mix or blend.
155. To make clean.
156. Gerard, 1434.

157. Dioscorides, Book 1, 86.

158. Ibid., 37.

159. In the Letters and Papers of Henry VIII an itemized list of the treatments and items made for Henry and his immediate household by his Gentlemen Apothecary. For the months of August, September, October and November, 273 items were made. December, the month before his death had close to as many items made as three of the previous months.

160. Glister (Glyster) a liquor made sometime with sodden flesh, sometime with decoction of herbs or other things, which by a Pipe is conveyed into the lower parts of the body.

161. *Letters and Papers, Foreign and Domestic, Henry VIII, Volume 14 Part 2*, 153.

162. "Hampton Court Palace".

163. "Ordinances for the household made at Eltham in the XVIIth year of King Henry VIII A.D. 1526", 174 in Nichols' *A collection of ordinances and regulations for the government of the royal household, made in divers reigns. From King Edward III. to King William and Queen Mary. Also receipts in ancient cookery.*

164. Bullein, "The Booke of Simples", Fol. 47.

165. Glyster, Glister, and Clyster all mean enema.

166. Bullein, "The Booke of Compoundes", Fol. 21.

167. Dioscorides, Book 1, 41.

168. Dioscorides, Book 2, 263.

169. Ibid.

170. Schilling and Webb.

171. Malik and Muller.

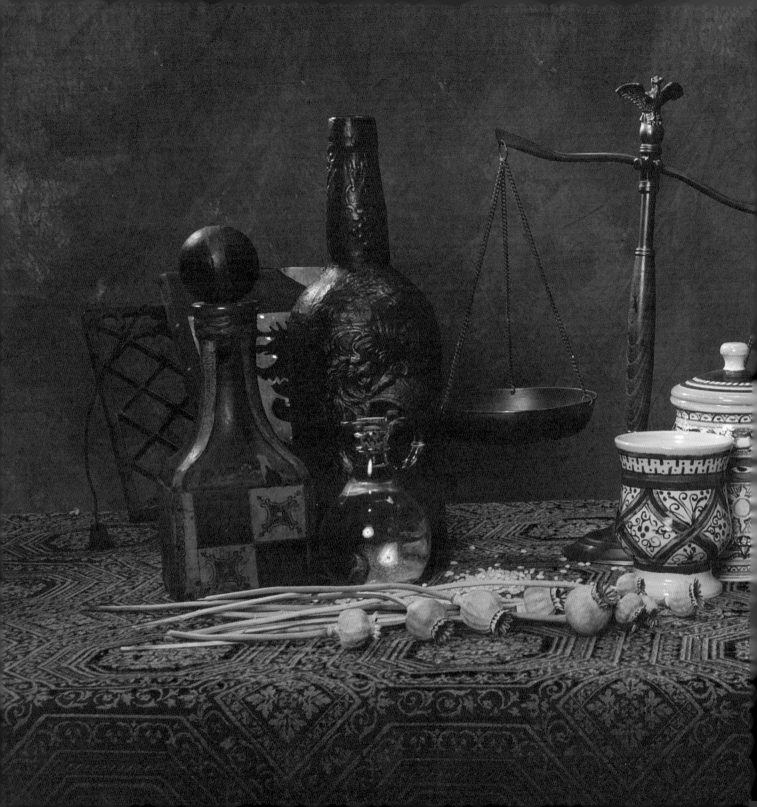

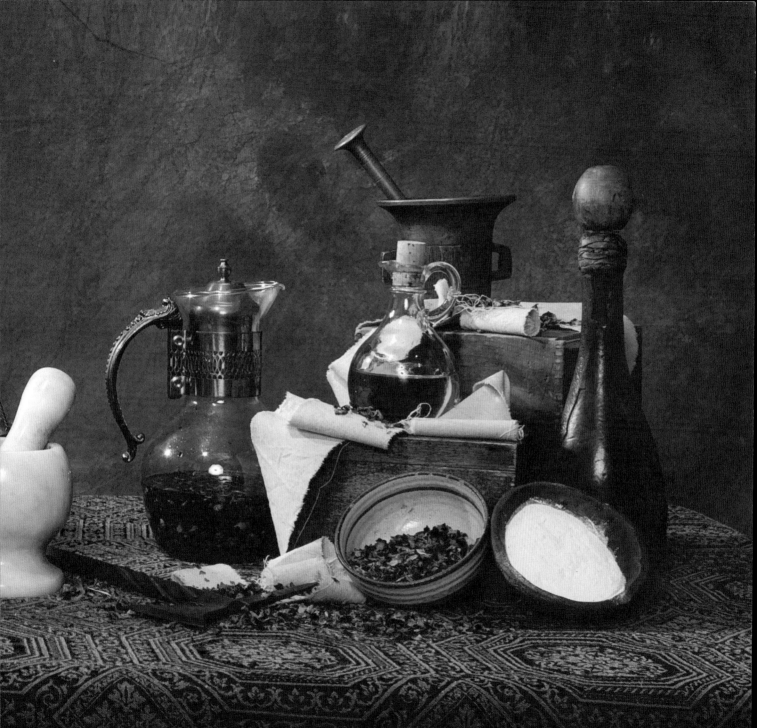

Historical Fiction

Falling Pomegranate Seeds - **Wendy J. Dunn**
Struck With the Dart of Love - **Sandra Vasoli**
Truth Endures - **Sandra Vasoli**
Phoenix Rising - **Hunter S. Jones**
Cor Rotto - **Adrienne Dillard**
The Raven's Widow - **Adrienne Dillard**
The Claimant - **Simon Anderson**
The Colour of Poison - **Toni Mount**
The Colour of Gold - **Toni Mount**
The Colour of Cold Blood - **Toni Mount**
The Colour of Betrayal - **Toni Mount**
The Colour of Murder - **Toni Mount**
The Colour of Death - **Toni Mount**
The Tudor Colouring Book - **Ainhoa Módenes**
The Wars of the Roses Colouring Book - **Debra Bayani**

Non Fiction History

The Turbulent Crown - **Roland Hui**
Anne Boleyn's Letter from the Tower - **Sandra Vasoli**
Queenship in England - **Conor Byrne**
Katherine Howard - **Conor Byrne**
Jasper Tudor - **Debra Bayani**
Tudor Places of Great Britain - **Claire Ridgway**
Illustrated Kings and Queens of England - **Claire Ridgway**
A History of the English Monarchy - **Gareth Russell**
The Fall of Anne Boleyn - **Claire Ridgway**
George Boleyn: Tudor Poet, Courtier & Diplomat - **Ridgway & Cherry**
The Anne Boleyn Collection - **Claire Ridgway**
The Anne Boleyn Collection II - **Claire Ridgway**
Two Gentleman Poets at the Court of Henry VIII - **Edmond Bapst**

Children's Books

All about Richard III - **Amy Licence**
All about Henry VII - **Amy Licence**
All about Henry VIII - **Amy Licence**
Tudor Tales William at Hampton Court - **Alan Wybrow**

PLEASE LEAVE A REVIEW

If you enjoyed this book, *please* leave a review at the book seller where you purchased it.
There is no better way to thank the author and it really does make a huge difference!
Thank you in advance.

Printed in Great Britain
by Amazon